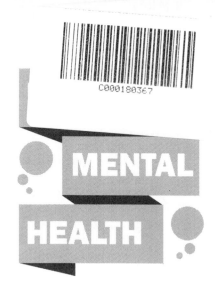

MENTAL
HEALTH

MEETING
THE MENTAL
HEALTH NEEDS
OF LEARNERS 11–18 YEARS

POSITIVE MENTAL HEALTH

This new series of texts presents a modern and comprehensive set of evidence-based strategies for promoting positive mental health in schools. There is a growing prevalence of mental ill health among children and young people within a context of funding cuts, strained services and a lack of formal training for teachers. The series recognises the complexity of the issues involved, the vital role that teachers play, and the current education and health policy frameworks in order to provide practical guidance backed up by the latest research.

Our titles are also available in a range of electronic formats. To order, or for details of our bulk discounts, please go to our website www.criticalpublishing.com or contact our distributor, NBN International, 10 Thornbury Road, Plymouth PL6 7PP, telephone 01752 202301 or email orders@nbninternational.com.

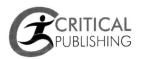

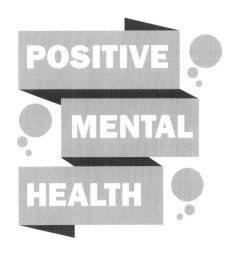

MEETING THE MENTAL HEALTH NEEDS

OF LEARNERS 11–18 YEARS

Jonathan Glazzard and Kate Bancroft

First published in 2018 by Critical Publishing Ltd

British Library Cataloguing in Publication Data
A CIP record for this book is available from the British Library

ISBN: 978-1-912508-12-9

This book is also available in the following e-book formats:

MOBI ISBN: 978-1-912508-13-6
EPUB ISBN: 978-1-912508-14-3
Adobe e-book ISBN: 978-1-912508-15-0

The rights of Jonathan Glazzard and Kate Bancroft to be identified as the Authors of this work have been asserted by them in accordance with the Copyright, Design and Patents Act 1988.

Cover and text design by Out of House Limited
Project Management by Out of House Publishing Solutions
Printed and bound in Great Britain by 4edge, Essex

Critical Publishing
3 Connaught Road
St Albans
AL3 5RX

www.criticalpublishing.com

Paper from responsible sources

✛ CONTENTS

✛ MEET THE SERIES EDITOR AND AUTHORS

JONATHAN GLAZZARD

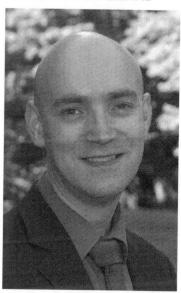

KATE BANCROFT

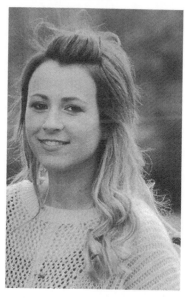

Jonathan Glazzard is series editor for *Positive Mental Health*. He is Professor of Teacher Education at Leeds Beckett University and also the professor attached to the Carnegie Centre of Excellence for Mental Health in Schools. He teaches across a range of QTS and non-QTS programmes and is an experienced teacher educator.

Kate Bancroft is a lecturer and course leader for BA (Hons) Childhood Studies at Leeds Beckett University. Her background is in secondary school teaching. She worked in four different secondary schools across Leeds, Halifax and Bradford and her roles included pastoral leader, head of department, head of faculty and assistant headteacher.

✛ INTRODUCTION

The Ministerial foreword to the government response to the consultation on the Green Paper *Transforming Children and Young People's Mental Health Provision*, published in December 2017 (Department for Education and Department of Health, 2017, p 3), states that:

Childhood should be the happiest time in a person's life, yet for thousands of children who develop mental illness in childhood or adolescence, the reality can be very different. One in ten (around 850,000) children and young people have a diagnosable mental health condition. These illnesses can have a devastating impact on their physical health, their relationships and their future prospects. The challenge often extends into a person's adult life, with half of all mental health conditions beginning before the age of 14.

Mental illness in young people appears to be increasing. We know that there is a link between social deprivation and mental ill health. We also know that adverse childhood experiences, including abuse, neglect and insecure attachments with primary caregivers contribute to poor mental health. However, school factors also play a role. Young people are learning at a time when expectations and pressures on them have never been higher. The 'knowledge-rich curriculum' has placed increased academic demands on students. Examination stress has increased; assessment through coursework has diminished in favour of terminal examinations that test students' abilities to recall subject content.

Young people are worried about what their futures will look like. The economy is unstable and jobs are not guaranteed. Higher education is a costly investment, to which some young people cannot financially commit. Family contexts, particularly those that are financially deprived, can be challenging for young people and relationships between young people and parents can be volatile when parents experience stress or have their own mental health needs.

The growth of social media in recent years has resulted in young people becoming addicted to their phones. Cyberbullying, body-image concerns

1

related to social media use and fear of missing out can result in the development of mental ill health. The pressure to share personal data and to respond instantly to messages can also place young people under stress.

Given this context, it is no surprise that young people are anxious, stressed and depressed. Anxiety, stress and depression can lead to self-harm and self-harm can lead to attempted suicide. Schools can do a great deal to support young people's mental health needs but it is not realistic to expect schools do this alone. Teachers are not in a position to diagnose a mental health need. However, they can identify warning signs that may warrant a referral. Support from external professional services and parents is vital if young people are to gain the support they need quickly. Currently, it is too difficult to gain a successful referral to child and adolescent mental health services. These services are at breaking point; they are overstretched and waiting times are too long. Ultimately, the responsibility falls to schools to address young people's mental health. However, education professionals are not health professionals and the primary role of the school is to promote learning. Despite this, the reality is that unless mental health needs are addressed this will have a detrimental effect on young people's academic development in school.

This book introduces you to the common mental health needs that you will experience in secondary schools. In each chapter, we outline the nature of the need and introduce strategies that schools can use to support young people with mental ill health.

Jonathan Glazzard and Kate Bancroft

✚ CHAPTER 1

FACTORS THAT PUT YOUNG PEOPLE AT RISK

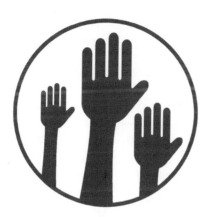

PROFESSIONAL LINKS

This chapter addresses the following:

- The Teachers' Standards (2011) state that a teacher must have a secure understanding of how a range of factors can inhibit pupils' ability to learn, and how best to overcome these (TS5, p 11).

- The Teachers' Standards state that a teacher is expected to demonstrate consistently high standards of personal and professional conduct (Part 2, p 14).

CHAPTER OBJECTIVES

By the end of this chapter you will understand:

+ risk factors within the school;
+ risk factors within the community;
+ risk factors within the family;
+ risk factors within the young person.

INTRODUCTION

This chapter introduces you to some of the critical factors that influence young people's mental health. Some of these factors are easier to control than others in your role as a teacher. You may not be able to mitigate factors which arise in the family or community, but you will be able to influence what happens in school and particularly within your own classroom. It is important to understand that several risk factors may be interrelated and therefore it may be difficult to attribute a single factor to a young person's mental health. As a teacher it is important that you try to understand what is causing a young person to have poor mental health. You will then be in a better position to decide whether you can influence the factor(s) to support the young person. It is also important to understand that 'within child' factors may have a social, cultural or environmental origin. For example, a child's poor self-concept or self-esteem may have been caused by factors in the school, community and/or the family, which may result in a poor sense of self. This chapter provides you with advice on what you can do to alleviate risk factors in your role as a teacher.

RISK FACTORS IN THE SCHOOL

Young people's mental health can be influenced by multiple factors in school. As a teacher, you can directly eradicate some of these factors in your own classroom. However, some risk factors within the school will require direct intervention by the senior leadership team.

THE SOCIAL AND EMOTIONAL ENVIRONMENT IN SCHOOL

Schools that have a positive culture promote a sense of belonging for all members of the school community. Within your classroom and in the wider school environment, it is important that you promote positive relationships between young people, adults, and between young people and adults. Positive relationships are rooted in mutual respect, empathy, dignity and a sense of feeling valued. As a teacher, you have a responsibility to model and promote these attributes. Some young people will demonstrate these attributes instinctively, but others will need encouragement to learn how to treat other people. In your classroom you can promote these values through your own interactions with the young people. Positive interactions might include:

+ smiling;

+ thanking young people and adults for their contributions;

+ listening without interruption;

+ demonstrating empathy when someone is distressed;

+ using praise and rewards;

+ rewarding effort as well as achievement;

+ promoting a 'can-do' culture;

+ recognising all achievements, however small;

+ using positive body language;

+ enabling all young people to recognise that they have strengths and talents.

You can directly teach young people about developing positive interactions with others in lessons by insisting that young people treat each other with respect, listen to the views of others and value diversity.

As a teacher, you have a duty to develop in young people a positive sense of self. It is important that you promote a positive climate in the classroom rather than promoting a climate of fear. Young people should never be afraid of trying things and getting them wrong. Additionally, young people should not be afraid to express their views, wishes or needs. It is important to empower young people to have a voice and to teach them how to respond appropriately to their peers in situations where someone makes a mistake or is distressed. You can do this by promoting a team spirit and by helping young people to recognise that they are part of a learning community in which everyone works together to help each other. Developing collaboration through group work in lessons is an effective tool for promoting these skills.

You will also need to consider your interactions with other adults in the room. As a role model you will need to demonstrate that you value the teaching assistant(s) and they will need to demonstrate that they value you. In addition, your interactions with parents should be respectful, even though you may have little contact with parents in secondary schools. It is critical that you treat parents with respect and dignity, even when they do not demonstrate these attributes towards you. This is perhaps one of the most difficult skills to demonstrate, particularly when parents may be angry with you, upset or distressed. You are the professional and it is important that you can remain calm and respectful consistently. It is also important to try to understand that some parents lead complex lives in challenging circumstances. Negative parental interactions towards you may not be personal. They may be a product of adverse circumstances that they have experienced, and you happen to be in the firing line! The same is also true for young people. If parents model inappropriate interactions with you in front of young people, your interactions with them need to be positive and calm so that young people observe appropriate ways of responding to others. They may not observe this at home. Obviously, if you are being threatened or abused you retain the right to terminate the conversation by asking the parent to leave in a polite way and requesting a follow-up appointment when they are calm.

TEACHER–PUPIL RELATIONSHIPS

The relationships that you form with young people are critical to their developing sense of self. You have a duty to form positive relationships with all young people and you will find this easier in cases where young people demonstrate positive attributes towards you. However, it can be more challenging to develop positive relationships with some young people. These include those who:

+ are disrespectful towards you;

+ demonstrate poor classroom behaviour;

+ demonstrate negative interactions with their peers;

+ demonstrate limited effort or lack motivation.

You will need to try to understand the causes of these negative behaviours so that you can support young people's development. For example, young people may demonstrate limited effort in lessons because they have a poor sense of self. If you recognise this, you can then focus on enhancing their self-concept and self-esteem. Poor behaviour is often an attempt to communicate an unmet need. Some young people may have disrupted, insecure or broken attachments with their parents or carers and this may affect their behaviour in the classroom. Understanding the causes of classroom behaviour will help you to demonstrate empathy towards the young person and to respond to them positively. As a teacher you cannot 'give up' on any young person. You should believe that fundamentally there are good characteristics within everyone and that some young people simply require additional support to demonstrate these characteristics. You can support young people to recognise that they are good at something. You can help them to realise that they can have a positive future. You can catch them being good and you can reward them. You can build their sense of self. You can help them to realise that they might find an aspect of learning difficult right now but eventually they will be able to grasp it. Believing in them is one of the most powerful things that you can do as a teacher.

CRITICAL QUESTIONS

You will need to consider how you interact with young people. The following questions should support you to do this.

+ Are you consistently positive with all young people?

+ Do you respond in different ways to different young people?

+ Are you consistently calm in the classroom, even in challenging situations?

+ Do you value young people's achievements?

+ Do you reflect on your own teaching when young people fail to understand something?

+ Do you believe that all young people have positive traits?

+ Do you believe that all young people have potential?

+ Do you believe that there should always be consequences to poor behaviour?

CURRICULUM, TEACHING AND LEARNING

The curriculum should be carefully planned and structured so that all pupils are explicitly taught about wellbeing. Developing young people's mental health literacy is essential so that they can understand how to care for their own wellbeing. Additionally, young people need to be taught how their own interactions towards others can influence the wellbeing of other people. In secondary schools, a mental health curriculum should typically cover a range of themes including how to manage stress, anxiety and depression, self-harm, overcoming adversity, resilience and substance abuse. This is not an exhaustive list. It is important that young people understand that everyone has mental health. It is also important that they recognise that mental health falls along a continuum which ranges from positive mental health to mental illness and that people's mental health can fluctuate depending on life events. Even in secondary schools there may be some reluctance to use the terms 'mental health' or 'mental illness' with young people. This may be due to the belief that young people should be protected from discussions about mental health. However, it is attitudes like this that lead to the stigmatisation of mental health. It is important to normalise and de-stigmatise mental health so that young people do not grow up to believe that mental health is something that should not be discussed.

Lack of curriculum breadth and balance can also affect young people's mental health (House of Commons Education Committee, 2018). The focus on the academic curriculum in secondary schools can lead to the development of a poor self-concept and reduced confidence, particularly for those who find these subjects more difficult or less interesting. Young people need access to a rich curriculum that includes vocational and technical subjects, sport, science, music, the creative and performing arts, and the humanities. Providing a curriculum that offers breadth to all young people will enable the development of their talents. This will boost their confidence and will help to develop a positive sense of self. Lack of curriculum choice in secondary schools can result in disengagement and a poor sense of wellbeing.

CRITICAL QUESTIONS

+ What are your views on using the terms 'mental health' and 'mental illness' with young people?

+ Why do you think mental health has been stigmatised in the past?

+ What are your views on introducing young people to themes such as depression, anxiety and stress?

STUDENT VOICE

Giving young people a voice helps to empower them. It builds their confidence and fosters a sense of belonging. These are vital for their well-being. Historically, schools and society in general did not allow young people to have a voice. However, views on voice have changed significantly. Young people are now viewed as social agents. This means that they should be viewed as confident individuals who can express their views. Your school should have mechanisms for eliciting student voice. These might include student councils, which represent the views of all young people in the school. In your classroom you can use a range of approaches to facilitate student voice. These include:

+ a post box for young people to post confidential notes to an adult;

+ involving young people in decisions about what they want to learn by involving them in curriculum planning;

+ providing young people with opportunities to review their own learning and behaviour through termly student consultation meetings with an adult;

+ giving young people opportunities to set their own targets;

+ providing young people with opportunities to make decisions about classroom resources which need to be purchased;

+ introducing a 'you said, we did' system so that young people can recognise what influence they have had in their classroom;

+ developing a pupil voice wall.

It is critical to ensure that all young people are provided with a voice, including those with speech, language and communication difficulties. For young people with no verbal communication, you will need to develop ways of providing them with an opportunity to express their views. One way of doing this is to use signs, photographs or symbols. These can be presented to young people so that they can make a choice by pointing to their preference. Some young people may lack confidence to express their views in a larger group but may be willing to express their views in a smaller group. Some young people may not be confident expressing their views to the teacher or to the class but may be confident in expressing their views to a peer, teaching assistant or other adult. Some may be reluctant to express their views orally but may find it easier to express their views in writing or in pictorial form. As a teacher, you need to find different ways of giving young people a voice so that barriers to expressing their views are removed.

SOCIAL CONTEXTS: PEER INFLUENCES

Bullying and discrimination can have a detrimental impact on young people's mental health. Your school will have a whole-school policy for addressing bullying and it is important that you familiarise yourself with this policy. There is a wide range of types of bullying, including physical and verbal bullying and cyberbullying. Sexual harassment is also a form of bullying because it constitutes an abuse of power and is designed to undermine the victim. This can include verbal comments and unwelcome and inappropriate forms of contact.

Micro-forms of aggression targeted at individuals also constitute bullying. These include laughing, whispering or making jokes about someone. Young people in secondary schools may also become victims of online bullying. If you identify bullying in school, you have a responsibility to address it. All forms of bullying should be challenged because they have no place in a school. Your school policy will guide you on how to respond to incidents of bullying.

Addressing bullying through tackling it when it occurs is essential, but reactive. Teachers also need to be proactive by educating all young people about the various forms of bullying and the impact that it can have on the victims. Schools should develop an anti-bullying curriculum which addresses all types of bullying. This curriculum should teach young people how to respond if they witness bullying so that young people do not become bystanders.

Discrimination is a deliberate attempt to treat someone less favourably than others. In secondary schools this might involve subtle tactics such as ignoring someone or excluding them from participating in an activity. Schools have a legal duty to prevent all forms of discrimination. In England, the Equality Act, 2010, makes it illegal for schools to discriminate of the grounds of protected characteristics. These include sex, race, disability, religion or belief, sexual orientation, gender reassignment and pregnancy or maternity. Examples of unlawful discrimination include:

+ a teacher refusing to allow a specific pupil to make contributions to questions and discussions in class because they have a protected characteristic;

+ boys and girls not being given the same curriculum opportunities;

+ treating girls more favourably than boys or vice versa;

+ providing unequal access to resources for boys and girls;

+ refusing to admit a young person to a school because their parents are lesbian or because they have a protected characteristic.

Some young people may not intend to bully or discriminate but may use language which is perceived to be discriminatory. One example of this includes the casual use of 'that is so gay' in secondary schools. The association of the word 'gay' with 'rubbish' is deeply problematic and although an individual may not have intended to cause hurt, it may not be perceived in the same way by young people who identify as lesbian, gay, bisexual or transgender. In secondary schools, many young people are aware of their sexual orientation and therefore the casual use of phrases like this can result in psychological distress. Schools should challenge language which is intended as 'banter' and should educate all young people about the damaging effects of it.

It is important to provide opportunities for victims of bullying and discrimination to sit down with perpetrators to resolve conflicts. Too often, well-meaning teachers intervene and make all the decisions in cases where young people are being treated less favourably. Restorative approaches which require perpetrators and victims to talk through conflict are particularly effective and provide young people with ownership. It can be highly effective for a perpetrator to listen to the effects of bullying or discrimination from the victim's perspective. It is also useful to ask the perpetrator how they intend to solve the problem. Teachers tend to tell the 'bully' how to respond in situations like this but it is the perpetrator's responsibility to solve the problem that they have created.

Schools should have processes for logging all bullying incidents to help them to identify patterns. It is good practice to note:

+ the type of bullying which took place;

+ the context surrounding incidents: what was happening at the time;

+ when the incident took place, including times of the day, days of the week;

+ the frequency of incidents;

+ the triggers;

+ the details of follow-up discussions and details of how incidents were followed up;

+ the consequence(s) applied and their effectiveness.

This checklist will help you to identify the factors that may be causing the young person to behave in specific ways. You need to note the context in which the bullying takes place because it is possible that specific triggers might be responsible and if you know what they are then you can try to eradicate them. It is important to recognise that all young people can change their behaviour and that, with education, support and encouragement, young people can cease bullying behaviours. The bully needs as much support as the victim to help them change their behaviour. You need to try to understand the factors that might contribute to a young person's behaviour. The following questions will help you.

CRITICAL QUESTIONS

+ Does the young person have a poor sense of self? If so, what factors may have caused this?

+ Is the young person able to identify their strengths?

+ Are parent-child interactions positive?

+ Has the young person formed secure attachments with their parents?

+ How stable is the young person's home life?

+ What behaviours does the young person witness in the family?

+ Is the young person neglected or being bullied by others?

+ Has the young person formed secure friendships in school?

These questions will help you to understand the young person's behaviour. While you are not able to influence some of these factors, they will help you to understand the young person and empathise with them.

This knowledge will support you in responding positively to the 'bully' as well as to the victim.

- One in ten young people has a diagnosable mental health disorder, the equivalent of approximately three students in every classroom.

- One in five young adults has a diagnosable mental health disorder.

- Half of all mental health problems manifest by the age of 14, with 75 per cent by age 24.

- Almost one in four children and young people shows some evidence of mental ill health, including anxiety and depression.

- In 2015, suicide was the most common cause of death for both boys (17 per cent of all deaths) and girls (11 per cent) aged between 5 and 19 years.

- One in 12 young people self-harms at some point in their lives, although there is evidence that this could be a lot higher. Girls are more likely to self-harm than boys.

(Young Minds: https://youngminds.org.uk)

Negative peer influences can have a detrimental effect on young people's wellbeing. These include:

+ bullying, harassment and discrimination;

+ being excluded from social groups;

+ being inducted into risk-taking behaviours by peers.

Secondary schools should provide a curriculum which addresses themes such as drug and alcohol abuse, other forms of substance abuse, sexual harassment, responsible use of social media, cyberbullying and manipulation or coercion within friendships. Sudden changes of behaviour may indicate that a young person has been subjected to negative peer influences. When you notice that there is a problem you will need to address it by following the school's policies. However, it is also important in the curriculum to teach young people to come forward if they observe negative peer interactions.

In secondary schools some young people may be worried about coming forward for fear of repercussions. In these instances, you may decide to preserve the young person's anonymity to limit the possibility of repercussions. However, the school policy should also clearly detail any consequences for the perpetrator in cases where negative peer influences continue.

SOCIAL ISOLATION

Social networks are essential to good mental health. Young people need to form friendships to engender a sense of belonging in school. Young people who are socially isolated may not form friendships easily and this can impact detrimentally on self-concept, self-esteem and confidence. Some young people are more at risk than others of experiencing social isolation. These include:

+ those with special educational needs and/or disabilities;

+ travellers, refugees and those seeking asylum;

+ those who identify as lesbian, gay, bisexual or transgender;

+ looked-after young people;

+ those who are neglected;

+ those who arrive at a school part-way through the year.

This is not an exhaustive list. As a teacher you should plan frequent opportunities for young people to work in pairs and small groups. This is an effective pedagogical approach that is theoretically underpinned by social constructivist theory. However, placing young people in fixed groups limits the opportunities for developing social relationships. Young people need regular opportunities to work with different young people. Adopting a flexible approach to grouping will ensure that young people are able to talk to and work with different young people in the classroom. Pedagogically, it is also good practice. Placing young people in a fixed ability group within one subject cannot meet their needs all the time because young people will demonstrate varying levels of abilities in different strands of that subject. Additionally, young people's abilities rapidly change during the year so grouping arrangements should be sufficiently flexible to respond to this need.

If you notice that a young person is experiencing social isolation, you might try pairing them with a 'buddy' who can socialise with them at break times. Additionally, you could nominate a group of young people who can take responsibility for including a young person in their group when they are outside the classroom.

CRITICAL QUESTIONS

+ Some young people with autistic spectrum conditions experience difficulties with social interactions and social communication. What are your views on supporting these young people to develop social relationships?
+ What are the arguments for and against this?

THE POLITICAL CONTEXT: EXAM STRESS

Exam stress is evident within secondary schools. Young people take formal statutory tests at the end of Key Stages. GCSE and A-level examinations are particularly stressful for young people because they are 'high stakes'. The impact of standardised testing on those young people who do not achieve the expected standard is significant and should not be underestimated. These young people can experience a poor sense of self and reduced confidence, and they can start to disengage from education. The reduction of coursework and renewed emphasis on terminal examinations at GCSE has also increased levels of stress, anxiety and depression in young people. More challenging curriculum content and reduced curriculum choice has also had a negative impact on young people's mental health.

All teachers need to regularly assess young people to plan effectively for their next steps in learning. Assessment which promotes learning is usually conducted informally minute by minute within lessons and between lessons by marking students' work. The standardised tests serve a different purpose. They provide a summary of what young people know and can do at a specific point in time. They rarely aid lesson planning, but the results are used to determine the overall effectiveness of the school. School effectiveness in secondary schools is based on narrow performance indicators, including examination results and progress data. The tests provide evidence to support school accountability. If the results are good, schools can demonstrate to governors, parents, academy leaders, local authorities, Ofsted and the Department for Education that it is providing good value for money. The results are entered on league tables which rank schools from the best to the worst performing schools. Thus, these assessments are high stakes.

The problem with high-stakes testing is that young people are required to take formal assessments that are stressful and divorced from the usual learning context. Stress is placed on school leaders to obtain good results and this pressure is then transmitted down to teachers and often to young people. However, the assessments rarely provide teachers with additional information about what the young person knows and can do. Good teachers have this knowledge already through their continuing informal assessments. The tests simply enable a school to demonstrate that it is either performing or not. Young people are caught up in the accountability regime and those who do not meet the expected standards become victims of it. Young people place a significant amount of stress on themselves to perform well in terminal examinations and some parents also place pressure on their child to perform.

Standardised testing was first implemented in primary schools in 1988 through the Education Reform Act. Over the past three decades, the status of the tests has increased from low to high stakes. All governments have remained firmly committed to the tests, despite union opposition. While you will have no control in relation to administering the tests, you should try to keep the process 'low key' for the young people. The following advice will support you to achieve this.

+ Avoid transmitting your stress to the young people.

+ Remind young people that the tests are a partial assessment of what they know and can do – they have talents which you recognise which are not being tested.

+ Tell young people not to worry about examinations. They simply need to focus on doing their personal best and many people have been extremely successful in life regardless of how well they performed in their GCSEs.

+ Inform young people that the outcome of the tests will not determine their futures.

+ Teach young people some breathing exercises to aid anxiety and encourage them to use these during the assessments.

+ During examinations, ask young people to imagine taking the test in their favourite place.

+ If young people are feeling anxious, teach them some simple mindfulness techniques. You might want to try asking them to hold a raisin. Encourage them to feel it and smell it. Then ask them to put it in their mouths and to focus on only the raisin. Ask them to think about the texture and the flavour. Ask them to hold it in their mouths for one or two minutes before finally eating it.

CRITICAL QUESTIONS

+ What are your views on exam stress?

+ Do you agree that an element of stress or anxiety can be a positive thing?

FAMILY FACTORS

The Green Paper on mental health states that:

Adverse Childhood Experiences, such as trauma, poor attachment, parental alcohol and drug abuse, domestic violence, and so on, have a known and significant effect on the child's future mental well-being.

(House of Commons Education and Health and Social Care Committees, 2018, para 40)

Risk factors that detrimentally impact on young people's mental health include:

+ parental conflict;

+ family breakdown;

+ hostile or rejecting relationships;

+ abuse and neglect;

+ parental psychiatric distress;

+ parental criminality;

+ parental alcoholism;

+ death and loss;

+ young people moving into care, being fostered or adopted;

+ poverty, socioeconomic disadvantage or parental unemployment.

As a teacher, you will need to be aware of which young people in your class are experiencing these risk factors. Some of these young people may have been identified as having special educational needs. In these cases, the Special Educational Needs Coordinator may be aware of the risk factors and they may be able to share relevant information with you, particularly in cases where young people's learning and behaviour are being affected. However, some young people in these circumstances may not have special educational needs. You will need to be aware of changes of mood and behaviour that may be indicative of problems at home. Sometimes young people may alert you to situations at home, although this may be rare. If you suspect that a young person is being abused or neglected, you should always follow the guidance in your school's safeguarding policy. It is not acceptable to do nothing.

It is important that you provide a safe, nurturing environment for all young people, but particularly for young people who are experiencing adverse circumstances at home. The circumstances at home may result in the child demonstrating a poor sense of self, high levels of anxiety or stress, reduced confidence and disengagement in the classroom. Adverse circumstances at home can result in social, emotional and behavioural difficulties. Some young people who experience adverse circumstances may be operating at higher stages of cognitive development. If you notice that they are not making sufficient progress, this could indicate that the child might be experiencing problems at home. It is important not to jump to conclusions but if problems persist then you should discuss the next steps with senior teachers in your school. Young people from a range of social backgrounds may experience abuse, neglect, parental mental health issues and parental conflict. It is important not to assume that problems only occur in areas of social deprivation.

CASE STUDY

A secondary school had identified that a large proportion of parents had mental health needs. The school was situated in an area of high unemployment and many of the parents did not work. During the previous two years there had been a surge in the number of fathers committing suicide. Many of these cases had resulted from financial difficulties, including debt. Many of the parents were not productive during the day and spent their time drinking alcohol. The school developed several projects specifically aimed at improving the mental health of the parents. They ran a series of workshops which addressed the following themes:

+ debt management;

+ applying for jobs;

+ writing a CV;

+ voluntary work in the community;

+ stress management;

+ mindfulness and relaxation;

+ services in the community that can help.

The sessions were popular because the school provided a free lunch for those who attended.

CRITICAL QUESTIONS

+ Do you agree with the approach adopted by this school?

+ What are the advantages and disadvantages of offering workshops to parents?

ATTACHMENT

John Bowlby developed a theory of attachment. He argued that a strong attachment to a primary caregiver, usually the mother, provides security and that the early bonds that young people form with their caregivers have a lasting impact that continues throughout life. Bowlby was particularly interested in separation anxiety, which results from young people being separated from their primary caregivers. Secure attachments are demonstrated when young people become distressed when they are separated from their caregiver but express joy when they are reunited with them. Avoidant attachments are demonstrated when young people avoid feeling an attachment towards their primary caregivers. Bowlby's work was developed further by Mary Ainscow (Bretherton, 1992).

CRITICAL QUESTIONS

+ What are the criticisms of attachment theory?

+ What are the stages of attachment?

+ What are the types of attachment?

+ How can attachment affect young people's mental health?

CASE STUDY

CULTURAL CONTEXTS

A large secondary school in a multicultural community introduced a mental health programme for students in Years 7 and 8. many of the parents were extremely resistant to this programme. Perspectives on mental health vary across families, ethnicities, cultures and countries. For these parents, their cultural and religious values had influenced their beliefs about mental health and many of them held negative perceptions about mental illness. A group of parents signed a petition to stop the programme being introduced and this was sent to the Chair of Governors. One of the parents contacted Ofsted to make a formal complaint about the school. Some of the parents withdrew their children from lessons.

CRITICAL QUESTIONS

+ What factors may have shaped the views of these parents?

+ Imagine that you hold the position of Chair of Governors. What would your response have been to the petition?

+ Should the school abandon the programme?

+ How might the school work with parents to help them understand the importance of this programme?

+ Does the school have a role to play in influencing religious and cultural values?

COMMUNITY FACTORS

A range of risk factors that have their origins in the community can have a detrimental impact on young people's mental health. These include:

+ disasters;

+ accidents;

+ war;

+ other significant events;

+ homelessness;

+ socioeconomic disadvantage.

Socioeconomic disadvantage acts as a psychosocial stressor and can work through poor housing and unsafe neighbourhoods to negatively impact young people's mental health and wellbeing. It limits the ability of young people to participate in activities with their peers. It is associated with worse parental mental, which is, in turn, a strong risk factor for poor child mental health and wellbeing.

(Education Policy Institute, 2018)

⏺ Socioeconomically disadvantaged young people and adolescents are two to three times more likely to develop mental health problems.

⏺ Child poverty is projected to increase to 37 per cent by 2022.

(Education Policy Institute, 2018)

WITHIN-PERSON FACTORS

Risk factors within the young person can have a detrimental effect on their mental health. These factors may include:

+ genetic factors;

+ low confidence;

+ low self-esteem;

+ academic failure;

+ learning difficulties.

Some of these 'within-person' factors may have been caused by school, family and community factors. Low self-esteem might be a result of insecure attachments between the young person and their primary caregiver. Learning difficulties may be biological but may have been inherited from parents. Academic failure may be a result of socioeconomic deprivation or it may have been caused by factors within the school. Environmental factors can influence the architecture in the brain. The brain is malleable and is highly responsive to environmental effects. As a teacher, you can influence many of the factors within the young person through:

+ developing their self-concept and self-esteem;

+ listening to young people's perspectives;

+ developing their confidence;

+ providing access to high-quality teaching which meets their needs;

+ providing a positive, nurturing environment in the classroom to enable the young person to thrive;

+ developing positive relationships with young people.

SUMMARY

This chapter has focused on the risk factors in school that affect young people's mental health, because this is where you can have the greatest influence as a teacher. You can control what happens in school, but there is no guarantee that you can influence what happens in the home or in the community. However, this does not mean that you cannot exert some influence. Risk factors rarely occur in isolation. They are complex and interrelated. Being aware of the risk factors will enable you to identify young people who may be at risk of developing mental health problems.

CHECKLIST

This chapter has addressed:

✓ the importance of providing a safe, positive and nurturing environment in school;

✓ the relationship between socioeconomic deprivation and young people's mental health;

✓ the relationship between secure early attachments with primary caregivers and young people's mental health.

FURTHER READING

Heaven, B (2012) *The Mental Health Handbook for Primary School: Raising Awareness of Mental Health Issues and How to Deal with Them.* Abingdon: Routledge.

Hollinsley, J (2018) *An Educator's Guide to Mental Health and Wellbeing in Schools.* Woodbridge: John Catt Educational.

✚ CHAPTER 2

IDENTIFYING AND SUPPORTING YOUNG PEOPLE WITH ANXIETY AND DEPRESSION

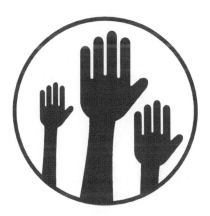

PROFESSIONAL LINKS

This chapter addresses the following topic:

⟠ The special educational needs and disabilities code of practice identifies mental health as a special need. Anxiety and depression are examples of mental health needs.

CHAPTER OBJECTIVES

By the end of this chapter you will understand:

+ the causes of anxiety and depression;

+ the signs of anxiety and depression;

+ ways of supporting young people with anxiety and depression.

INTRODUCTION

This chapter introduces you to the factors which can result in young people developing anxiety and depression. There is an established link between depression and self-harm and suicide, so it is important that it is taken seriously. The chapter covers different forms of anxiety and depression and introduces you to strategies that schools can use to support young people.

FACTORS THAT RESULT IN ANXIETY AND DEPRESSION

Anxiety and depression do not distinguish between age, background or social group. Most people experience anxiety and depression at some point in their lives. Experiences in life can trigger these emotions. Young people may demonstrate signs of anxiety and depression, but this does not necessarily indicate that they have a mental health disorder. It is usual to feel anxious when faced with a new or stressful situation. Younger children may be afraid of the dark. This does not mean that they have a mental health need. It is a normal reaction to feel sad in specific situations. It is typical to experience low mood from time to time. Anxiety and depression are part of typical childhood development. When the feelings are intense and persistent, this might indicate that there is a mental health need.

When depression and anxiety persist for long periods of time this may indicate that the young person may have a mental health need and may need support. This is pertinent when the anxiety and depression prevent the young person from participating fully in day-to-day activities.

Anxiety and depression may be caused by various factors. Some young people are concerned about their appearance. According to the Royal

Society for Public Health (2017), 'As many as nine in 10 teenage girls say they are unhappy with their body' (p 10). Social media use plays a part in some young people developing a 'compare and despair' attitude; they compare their appearance to digitally edited photographs of slender celebrities and this can result in low body esteem, which can be a cause of anxiety and depression in young people. This issue is not just pertinent to girls. Boys can also develop low body esteem after viewing images of well-toned muscular bodies. Advertisements and images on television, radio, in newspapers and magazines also play a role in young people developing body image issues.

There are other significant factors that can result in anxiety, stress and depression. Young people are under significant pressure in schools to perform well in their examinations. Teachers may transmit their own stress in relation to this directly to young people. Parental expectations also play a role in contributing to 'exam stress'. Additionally, young people also place significant pressure on themselves to perform well in exams. They face an uncertain future as competition for jobs is high. The unstable financial climate can also be a factor which causes young people to worry about their future. GCSE and A-level examinations have become more difficult as the emphasis on terminal exams, rather than course work, has resulted in increased pressure on young people to memorise subject content. Success is now largely determined by performance on the end of course examinations and this places undue stress on young people. The recent changes to the national curriculum have resulted in young people learning more complex subject content which can increase stress and reduce self-esteem.

Young people now live in a digital world where friendships and identities are played out over social media. Young people may experience pressure to respond instantly to messages or to accept 'friend' requests over social media. They may experience anxiety about being accepted into a social circle and this may be heightened by social media, through which young people form instant 'friendships'. Cyberbullying can result in stress, anxiety and depression. According to the Royal Society of Public Health:

Victims of bullying are more likely to experience low academic performance, depression, anxiety, self-harm, feelings of loneliness and changes in sleeping and eating patterns – all of which could alter the course of a young person's life as they undertake important exams at school or university.

(Royal Society of Public Health, 2017)

Young people may experience anxiety and depression because of their sexual or gender identity. According to the latest statistics from Stonewall, 84 per cent of young people who identify as transgender have self-harmed and 61 per cent of lesbian, gay and bisexual young people who are not transgender have self-harmed and 22 per cent have attempted to take their own life (Bradlow et al, 2017). Episodes of anxiety and depression may have been evident before the self-harm and attempted suicide took place.

Social deprivation is another contributing factor that can result in anxiety and depression. Young people from low income families may be worried about the financial circumstances in their family. Their parents may also be anxious and depressed about their financial situation and this worry can transfer to their children. The threat of homelessness or lack of food can cause anxiety and depression. Additionally, young people from all social backgrounds can experience abuse and neglect, which can result in anxiety and depression. The experience of living in an unhappy family or in a family where there is conflict can trigger depression. Parental separation and divorce can also be a trigger for depression. Domestic violence in the home can result in anxiety and depression and young people may start to fear for their own safety and for the safety of others in the family. A family member becoming ill can trigger depression. These issues can be evident in families from a range of social backgrounds; they are not solely evident in socially deprived families.

TYPES OF ANXIETY AND DEPRESSION

Anxiety and depression are often discussed interchangeably but they are quite different things. While depression is characterised by persistent low mood, anxiety is a form of stress that is not characterised by persistent low mood. For example, someone might be anxious about travelling on the motorway, but they may not experience low mood. However, the two are connected because anxiety can result in depression. A person may experience social anxiety. Consequently, they may avoid social situations and demonstrate signs of social withdrawal. Social withdrawal can result in depression because social connections can have a positive effect on a person's wellbeing.

Two important points to remember are that:

sion are not signs of weakness;

EXAM STRESS AND ANXIETY

It is normal to feel stressed and anxious about tests and examinations. This can be a good thing because it can prompt young people to work harder in preparation for the exam. Exam stress can be triggered when the amount of preparation or revision that needs to be done starts to feel overwhelming. Young people may also feel stressed or anxious about the content of the test. They may be worried that they will not be able to answer the questions. They may be anxious about the grade they might achieve, and they may start to worry that they will let other people down if they do not perform well in the exam. Exam stress and anxiety start to become a problem when these feelings become overwhelming and disproportionate. These feelings of stress and anxiety may result in them not preparing for the exam because they imagine that failure is inevitable. They may convince themselves that it is better not to revise than to put effort into preparing well only to end up failing. The feelings of stress and anxiety at the preparation stage may be so intense that the young person is then unable to concentrate on the revision. During the examination the feelings of stress and anxiety may be so intense that they prevent the young person from performing well. They may start to imagine during the exam that everyone else is doing much better than they are and these feelings may prevent them from concentrating on the exam itself, thus resulting in them not performing in line with their ability. After the examination, they may experience stress and anxiety about the grades they will achieve. This may prevent them from participating in other activities due to the persistent feelings of fear and worry.

Depression is characterised by intense low mood. Low mood is not a symptom of depression. Everyone experiences low mood from time to time. When someone is depressed, feelings of hopelessness, negativity and helplessness are persistent and intense. Fear of potential failure can result in young people becoming lethargic during exam periods. Young people may also demonstrate signs of depression after an exam. This may be triggered by their experience of the exam itself or in response to the grade they ultimately achieved. It is usual for everyone to experience a low mood when the grade achieved does not match the grade that was expected or even when the grade achieved does not match the grade that was desired. These situations can result in feelings of disappointment and low mood, but these feelings usually subside after a short time. When they persist for a long period of time this could indicate that the young person has a mental health need. When the feelings are disproportionate to the situation this could also indicate that the young person might have a mental health need, for example, if they feel that their life chances are ruined because they have not achieved the desired grade.

CRITICAL QUESTIONS

+ In what situations might stress and anxiety be beneficial?
+ What strategies might alleviate exam stress and anxiety?

SEPARATION ANXIETY

Separation anxiety arises when a young person is separated from their parents or guardians. The feelings of anxiety only subside when the young person is reunited with their parents. During the day when the young person is at school, they may demonstrate signs of anxiety. They may constantly worry about their parents when they are not with them. For example, they may worry about their parents' safety or well-being when they are separated from them. They may experience anxiety during the night when they cannot see their parents. These feelings of anxiety can have a detrimental impact on the young person's academic performance because their concentration during the school day can become impaired. The separation can also result in depression, which only subsides when the young person is with their parents. Their relationships and interactions with peers can also be affected.

GENERALISED ANXIETY DISORDER

Generalised anxiety disorder is a form of persistent anxiety which has been evident for six months. It is characterised by feelings of constant anxiety. A young person may be anxious about a specific situation but when that situation is resolved another situation arises which causes the young person to become anxious. The feeling of being anxious does not subside as new factors arise which cause the young person to become anxious. Generalised anxiety disorder is also characterised by disproportionate feelings of worry. For example, the young person may start to worry when a parent is late home from work. Rather than assuming that their parent is at work completing jobs, they may assume that they have been involved in an accident on the way home and that they are injured or have died. The first assumption to a situation may be negative rather than logically considered. They may jump to the worst possible conclusion.

SOCIAL PHOBIA

Young people (and adults) may demonstrate social phobia. This is characterised by a fear of social situations. Examples include:

+ fear of group tasks;

+ fear of going to parties or other social occasions;

+ fear of public speaking;

+ fear of introducing oneself in a social situation.

The reasons for social phobia may vary. Some people feel that they will be the 'centre of attention' in a social situation and they may dislike this feeling. They may prefer other people to be the focus of attention rather than the attention being focused on them. Social phobia can become a problem when it prevents individuals from participating in activities from which they might benefit. They may start to avoid social contact or they may avoid specific situations. Social withdrawal can also be a sign of depression. It can also limit people's opportunities.

CRITICAL QUESTIONS

+ What factors might result in young people developing social phobias?

+ What strategies can schools implement to support young people who experience social phobias?

SPECIFIC PHOBIAS

A specific phobia is an intense fear towards an object or situation. Examples include:

+ fear of going to the doctor;

+ fear of going to school: 'school phobia';

31

+ fear of animals;

+ fear of insects;

+ fear of extreme weather;

+ fear of travelling on an aeroplane.

This is not an exhaustive list. Do you have any specific phobias that are not identified on this list? Most people have specific dislikes. When the fear of something becomes disproportionate to the risk, it can be a sign of a specific phobia. For example, someone might think that an aeroplane will crash if they travel on it even though the risk is very low. When the fear of something prevents someone from participating in activities which are a normal part of day-to-day life this could suggest that there may be a mental health need that needs to be addressed.

CRITICAL QUESTIONS

+ What factors might result in young people developing school phobia?

+ What strategies can schools implement to support young people who experience school phobia?

MILD DEPRESSION

Mild depression is characterised by intense and persistent low mood that has a limited negative effect on a person's daily life. For example, a young person may demonstrate persistent low mood, which can affect their motivation. However, this does not necessarily prevent them from participating in activities.

MAJOR DEPRESSION

Major depression is characterised by intense and persistent low mood which interferes with an individual's daily life. This can prevent them from participating in activities which are a normal part of day-to-day life and from which they would benefit.

BIPOLAR DISORDER

Bipolar disorder is characterised by mood swings, which can be extreme. Moods can change from feeling 'high' where the individual feels extremely elated and indestructible, to 'lows' which are characterised by feelings of intense depression. During the lows, they may experience suicidal thoughts and feelings of complete despair or extreme lethargy. These feelings can affect their productivity.

SEASONAL AFFECTIVE DISORDER

Seasonal affective disorder is evident when a person's mood is affected by lack of daylight. It is associated with the start of winter and can last until spring when longer days bring more daylight. The condition is sometimes called 'winter blues'.

POSTNATAL DEPRESSION

Teenage mothers who are still at school may demonstrate signs of post-natal depression. This condition is not the same thing as experiencing the 'baby blues', which normally occur a few days after the birth of a child. It is characterised by intense and persistent low mood. It can leave new mothers feeling completely overwhelmed, inadequate and experiencing feelings of being unable to cope. It can also be characterised by mothers developing negative feelings towards their child.

IDENTIFYING ANXIETY AND DEPRESSION

Anxiety and depression affect people in different ways. Signs of depression may include:

+ *avoiding activities that were previously enjoyed;*

+ *withdrawal and social isolation: avoiding friends or social situations;*

+ *changes in sleeping pattern: sleeping more or sleeping less than usual;*

+ *changes in eating habits: eating more or eating less than usual or irregular eating;*

+ *feeling irritable, upset, miserable or lonely;*

+ *being self-critical;*

+ *feeling hopeless or losing interest;*

+ *signs of self-harm;*

+ *continual thinking about previous negative experiences;*

+ *feeling tired and showing signs of lethargy.*

(Young Minds, https://youngminds.org.uk)

Other signs of depression include:

+ *thoughts of suicide;*

+ *insomnia;*

+ *changes in mood;*

+ *changes in appetite or weight change;*

+ *restlessness.*

Signs of anxiety may include:

+ *feeling restless or agitated;*

+ *panic attacks;*

+ *having trouble concentrating;*

+ *tiredness due to lack of sleep;*

+ *excessive sweating;*

+ *shortness of breath;*

+ *dizziness;*

+ *heart palpitations.*

(MQ: www.mqmentalhealth.org)

CRITICAL QUESTIONS

+ Some young people do not demonstrate visible signs of anxiety and depression. How can schools identify young people with mental health needs where the signs are not visible?

+ When might you refer a young person to specialist mental health services for support?

SUPPORTING YOUNG PEOPLE WHO HAVE EXPERIENCED GRIEF OR LOSS

Young people can experience grief through the death of a parent, sibling, other family member or friend. They might also experience grief because of the death of a pet. Young people might grieve for friendships they once had and have now lost, especially if they have moved to a new school, town or country. Young people might feel a sense of loss if they have experienced permanent or temporary separation from their parents or other family members. They might also experience feelings of loss during times of transition; for example, when they move to a new class, school or even when they move home. Grief and loss might result in anxiety, depression or even conduct disorders.

In relation to grief you should not be afraid to use the word 'death'. You might say 'I was sorry to hear that your dog has died'. It is better to be honest with young people rather than trying to protect them from the truth. When young people return to school following the death of someone, it is important to establish a clear sense of routine and to treat them in the usual way. You could talk to selected peers about how they can support the young person when they return to school. It is a good idea to meet with the young person on the first day to ask them what support they would like from you or the school. Some young people will be happy with no additional support while others may welcome the opportunity to talk to an adult when they feel upset. Some young people may also need a quiet space to go to enable them to reflect when they feel this is necessary.

You should not expect the young person to grieve for a specific period. Some young people need longer than others to grieve. Others will appear to be coping but they may still be anxious, depressed or lonely. Sometimes, following a period of grief, a young person may appear to be coping well but something may trigger a memory or an emotion. This might be a birthday, a special occasion, a place or even a happy event which they wish the deceased person could share. You will need to be patient with the young person and reassure them that this is not something they should feel bad about.

Training peer ambassadors to be 'listening ears' may be a useful strategy. Some people may prefer to speak to another young person about how they are feeling rather than talking to an adult. If a young person experiences chronic grief, then they may need further therapeutic interventions from specialist staff such as counsellors. Chronic grief is grief that is persistent, and which prevents an individual from functioning normally in their day-to-day life.

EVIDENCE-BASED APPROACHES TO SUPPORT YOUNG PEOPLE

This section addresses evidence-based strategies which have been proven to be effective for young people with anxiety and depression.

COGNITIVE BEHAVIOUR THERAPY

Young people tend to be anxious or depressed because they have developed a complex system of beliefs that make them think that the world is unmanageable, dangerous or difficult. Cognitive behaviour therapy helps young people to change these beliefs. It empowers young people to take control of situations by unlearning negative associations. It must be delivered by a qualified practitioner.

SCHOOL-BASED COUNSELLING

There is evidence to suggest that targeted school-based interventions have led to improvements in wellbeing and mental health, yielding reduced levels of school exclusion and improved pupil attainment (Banerjee et al, 2014). Research indicates that school-based counselling is perceived by young people and pastoral care workers as a highly accessible, non-stigmatising and effective form of early intervention for reducing psychological distress (Cooper, 2009).

SCHOOL NURSE

Young people with a long-term health condition are at an increased risk of stress, anxiety and depression. The risk is greater during periods of transition, during examinations and during admission to hospital (Gray, 2010). The school nurse plays a vital role in supporting young people with long-term health conditions to manage their condition. In addition, the school nurse plays a vital role in minimising the risk of anxiety

36

and depression. The school nurse can play a critical role in delivering aspects of the mental health curriculum. They can teach young people strategies for managing stress, anxiety and depression and they can support teachers to more effectively meet the needs of young people with anxiety and depression.

PEER SUPPORT

Peer support has been defined as:

Using the knowledge, skills and experience of children and young people in a planned and structured way to understand, support, inform and help develop the skills, understanding, confidence and self-awareness of other children and young people with whom they have something in common.

(Street and Herts, 2005)

The evidence base for peer support schemes is inconclusive. The programmes can take a variety of forms, including:

+ one-to-one peer support;

+ group peer support;

+ online support;

+ informal drop-in sessions.

Where there is evidence that peer support is effective, the programmes are characterised by clear 'buy-in' from the school leadership team, a dedicated member of staff who is responsible for running the programme and systematic monitoring to ensure that the programme is running smoothly (Department for Education, 2017b).

Often, young people prefer to talk to their peers about how they feel rather than to an adult. Peer ambassadors or peer mentors can be matched with vulnerable students to take on the role of 'friendly listeners' (Department for Education, 2017a). The peer mentor might need to refer a case on to an adult if there is a concern for a young person's safety, so they cannot assure confidentiality. However, they should make it clear to the young person why information needs to be shared, what information will be shared and who it will be shared with. They will require training in confidentiality and how to listen and suspend judgement. They will also need training in how to ask good questions.

SOLUTION-FOCUSED COACHING

Some young people may benefit from a solution-focused approach. In this approach the 'coach' helps the young person to recognise their strengths and to imaging how they might achieve a better future for themselves. The role of the coach is not to tell the young person how to improve their life or situation but to guide them to identify their own solutions. Questions that might be asked include:

+ On a scale of 1–10 how would you rate your current level of depression?

+ What could you do that will help you to move down the scale?

+ What are you good at?

+ If you could imagine the best future for you, what does that look like? What will it take to get you there?

+ On a scale of 1–10, how anxious are you?

+ What would make you less anxious? How could you move down the scale?

The conversation is strengths based rather than adopting a deficit approach. It focuses on what the young person can do to make them feel better and to have a better future. It empowers the young person to take ownership of their own mental health by helping them to understand that they can control how they feel.

SIGNPOSTING FOR FURTHER ADVICE

Young people who experience anxiety can contact Anxiety UK directly (www. anxietyuk.org.uk). This organisation will sign post them in the direction of further support. Young people can email the following account to receive advice: support@anxietyuk.org.uk.

For help with depression, young people can contact ChildLine: www.childline.org.uk; freephone: 0800 1111.

Young people can also contact the Samaritans (www.samaritans.org).

Depression Alliance is a UK-based charity for sufferers of depression. Their website contains information about depression and they have details of local support groups available for sufferers (www.depressionalliance.org).

Mind is a national mental health charity which offers information on where to find support groups in the local area for a range of mental health and emotional issues. They also provide information on where to go for more help (www.mind.org.uk).

Before young people are signposted to external agencies, however, schools should signpost them to school-based services, such as the school counselling service or the wellbeing or pastoral team. Schools can also signpost young people to peer ambassadors who have received training to enable them to provide peer support.

- One in six young people will experience an anxiety condition at some point in their lives.

- Five people in your class may be living with anxiety.

- 13.3 per cent of 16–19 year-olds and 15.8 per cent of 20–24 year-olds have suffered from anxiety.

- 1.7 per cent of 16–19 year-olds and 2.2 per cent of 20–24 year-olds have suffered from a depressive episode.

(AnxietyUK, www.anxietyuk.org.uk)

Additionally:

- depression is thought to occur in about 1 to 3 per cent of children and young people.

(Royal College of Psychiatrists, www.rcpsych.ac.uk/healthadvice/ parentsandyouthinfo/youngpeople/depressioninyoungpeople.aspx)

Research [Sampasa-Kanyinga and Lewis, 2015] suggests that young people who are heavy users of social media – spending more than two hours per day on social networking sites such as Facebook, Twitter or Instagram – are more likely to report poor mental health, including psychological distress (symptoms of anxiety and depression).

(Royal Society for Public Health, 2017, p 8)

CASE STUDY

A secondary school identified several students who found it difficult to cope with silence. The teachers were worried that the students would not cope well during their GCSE examinations because they found it difficult to cope with silence. For some, silence caused them to become anxious. The school decided to introduce mindfulness sessions to help all Year 11 students to manage silence. The school wanted the students to feel more comfortable with silence. The sessions used calming music and visualisation methods as relaxation techniques. The room was dimmed and candles were lit. Students were taught how to control their breathing through breathing exercises as a tool for reducing anxiety. In some sessions, students had the opportunity to develop mindful eating using fruit. At the end of the sessions the students felt relaxed and calm. They looked forward to these daily sessions which took place immediately after lunch time. During their GCSE examinations mindfulness was used prior to each examination to help the students to relax and feel calm. The students used the breathing techniques they had developed during the mindfulness sessions during their exams.

- 20 per cent of adolescents may experience a mental health problem in any given year;
- 50 per cent of mental health problems are established by age 14 and 75 per cent by age 24;
- 10 per cent of children and young people (aged 5–16 years) have a clinically diagnosable mental problem;
- 70 per cent of children and adolescents who experience mental health problems have not had appropriate interventions at a sufficiently early age.

(Mental Health Foundation, www.mentalhealth.org.uk)

There is growing evidence linking social media use and depression in young people, with studies showing that increased use is associated with significantly increased odds of depression [Lin et al, 2016]. Using social media for more than two hours per day has also been independently associated with poor self-rating of mental health, increased levels of psychological distress and suicidal ideation [Sampasa-Kanyinga and Lewis, 2015].

(Royal Society for Public Health, 2017, p 8)

CASE STUDY

A secondary school introduced sessions on stress and anxiety as part of the curriculum. Students were taught to recognise the signs of stress, depression and anxiety and they were introduced to techniques for managing these. They were taught about the important role that physical activity can play in reducing depression, stress and anxiety. They watched videos of famous celebrities talking about their own experiences of stress, depression and anxiety. Some of these celebrities included famous male footballers. They learned about the importance of talking to others about their feelings.

CRITICAL QUESTIONS

+ Why do you think it was important to show videos of male celebrities?

+ Why might some males be more reluctant than females to talk about their mental health?

+ What might be the effects of 'bottling things up' rather than talking to others?

SUMMARY

This chapter has introduced you to the factors which may result in anxiety and depression. Additionally, it has introduced you to the signs of anxiety and depression so that you can identify young people with mental health needs. We have emphasised that anxiety and depression are not necessarily mental health disorders. They only become a disorder when the problems are persistent, severe and prevent individuals from participating in daily life. We have emphasised some evidence-based strategies that schools can adopt to support young people with anxiety and depression.

CHECKLIST

This chapter has addressed that:

✓ anxiety and depression are not signs of weakness;

✓ most people experience anxiety and depression;

✓ a degree of anxiety is helpful in enabling young people to achieve their goals.

FURTHER READING

Charlie Waller Memorial Trust. [online] Available at: www.cwmt.org.uk (accessed 9 August 2018).

Schab, L (2008) *Beyond The Blues: A Workbook to Help Teens Overcome Depression*. Oakland, CA: New Harbinger.

+ CHAPTER 3

IDENTIFYING AND SUPPORTING YOUNG PEOPLE WITH CONDUCT DISORDERS

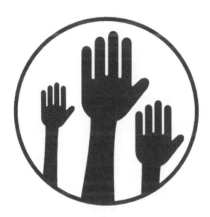

PROFESSIONAL LINKS

This chapter addresses the following:

- The special educational needs and disabilities code of practice identifies mental health as a special need. Anxiety and depression are examples of mental health needs.

- The *Teachers' Standards* (2011) place a duty on all teachers to meet the needs of all learners.

CHAPTER OBJECTIVES

By the end of this chapter you will understand:

+ what constitutes a conduct disorder;

+ the causes of conduct disorders;

+ how schools can support young people with conduct disorders.

INTRODUCTION

According to the report *Forgotten Children: Alternative Provision and the Scandal of Ever Increasing Exclusions*:

Mainstream schools should be bastions of inclusion, and intentionally or not, this is not true of all mainstream schools [p 3] ... An unfortunate and unintended consequence of the Government's strong focus on school standards has led to school environments and practices that have resulted in disadvantaged young people being disproportionately excluded, which includes a curriculum with a lack of focus on developing pupils' social and economic capital. There appears to be a lack of moral accountability on the part of many schools and no incentive to, or deterrent to not, retain pupils who could be classed as difficult or challenging [p 14].

(House of Commons Education Committee, 2018)

Teachers should never 'give up' on their students. In some cases, you may be the only sources of consistent support that a young person has. It is a sad reality that young people with conduct disorders are excluded from mainstream schools and placed in alternative provision. They are often marginalised in many ways, but the process of exclusion can lead to further marginalisation and it can cause mental ill health. We do not believe that exclusion should be viewed by schools as a way of solving a problem. It should only be used as a last resort. The reasons why young people develop conduct disorders vary. Schools need to invest in finding out the underlying causes of conduct disorders and developing interventions in partnership with young people, their parents and external agencies. This chapter is informed by the *Forgotten Children* report (House of Commons Education Committee, 2018). It explores some key issues and makes recommendations for the development of effective mainstream school practice.

FACTORS THAT RESULT IN CONDUCT DISORDERS

This section addresses the factors that may contribute to conduct disorders. These are divided into family, school and individual factors.

FAMILY FACTORS

Adverse childhood experiences can affect young people's behaviour. Young people who live in unsafe family environments are more likely to develop conduct disorders. Unsafe environments could include family environments where substance abuse, child abuse and neglect, and hostile relationships are evident, including parental conflict and domestic violence. A harsh and inconsistent parenting style or parental mental health problems can also result in conduct disorders. Young people who live in unsafe environments are more likely to be taken into care and more likely to be excluded from mainstream schools for conduct disorder than those who are not in care. Young people who continue to live in unsafe home environments where there is social services involvement are also more likely to develop conduct disorders and be excluded than those who live in safe households.

Young people who live in poverty are more likely to develop conduct disorders and be excluded than those who do not live in poverty. Child poverty is rising because of the slow economic recovery (Costa and Machin, 2015). Poverty can cause stress and volatile relationships in families and this can have a detrimental impact on young people's mental health and behaviour.

SCHOOL FACTORS

Several school factors can contribute to conduct disorders. These factors are identified in the *Forgotten Children* report (House of Commons Education Committee, 2018) and include the following considerations.

+ Lack of funding for pastoral support in schools can result in unmet needs. Cuts to school budgets in recent years because of the economic crisis have resulted in cuts to pastoral provision. This has meant that some young people do not receive the school-based intervention they need to support their behaviour.

+ Zero tolerance behaviour policies can result in young people disengaging from the mainstream education system. Some policies in schools are not flexible and this can result in young people being placed in isolation for relatively minor incidents. When this happens frequently it can have a detrimental effect on the young person's self-concept and this can then result in them developing conduct disorders that worsen and subsequently lead to temporary and permanent exclusions. Ironically, isolation can have the opposite effect to that intended. Rather than reducing behaviour problems, the young person's behaviour can worsen.

+ The narrow curriculum in secondary schools results in limited curriculum choice, which detrimentally impacts on the engagement of some young people. Young people who do not excel at English Baccalaureate subjects can then feel like failures and can develop a poor sense of self. This can detrimentally impact on their behaviour.

+ Some groups of young people are disproportionately represented in alternative provision. Black Caribbean pupils are disproportionally represented in alternative provision when the proportion of Black Caribbean pupils in the national population is considered. Other ethnic groups who are disproportionally represented in alternative provision include mixed ethnicity Black Caribbean and White pupils, Gypsy Roma heritage pupils and Irish traveller heritage pupils. Multiple vulnerabilities also exist. For instance, Black pupils are the ethnic group most likely to live in poverty with more than one in four eligible for free school meals (Shaw et al, 2016).

+ Young people with special educational needs and disabilities are more likely to develop conduct disorders and be excluded than those without such needs.

The over-representation of specific groups of young people in alternative provision indicates that mainstream schools are not consistently effective at supporting the most vulnerable students with conduct disorders. Young people with clinically diagnosed conduct disorders may also not be recognised by their mainstream schools as having a special educational need (Gill et al, 2017).

INDIVIDUAL FACTORS

The mental health and wellbeing of pupils is a factor that can result in the development of conduct disorders. Mental health issues can affect young people in different ways, including their abilities to cope with school, their attendance and their behaviour. These effects can result in a permanent or temporary exclusion into alternative provision, which can have a worsening effect on their mental health.

Boys are much more likely than girls to have a mental health disorder and a significant proportion of these needs will be in the form of conduct disorders. Girls with mental health problems are more likely to become withdrawn, demonstrate anxiety, depression, self-harm and are less likely to demonstrate aggression than boys.

Young people who leave primary schools with the lowest skill levels are most likely to demonstrate conduct disorders and be excluded from school (Gill et al, 2017). Data demonstrate that there is a strong relationship between a pupil's Key Stage 2 score, and the average number of fixed-period exclusions across their secondary school career (Strand and Fletcher, 2011; Gill et al, 2017).

TYPES OF CONDUCT DISORDERS

According to the Children's Society:

Conduct disorder is an emotional and behavioural condition that leads children and young people to act in a way that is disruptive and violent, and not follow rules.

(Children's Society, 2018)

Conduct disorders commonly coexist with other mental health problems. Conduct disorders include verbal and physical aggression, defiance and antisocial behaviour. They can have a detrimental impact on the academic achievement of themselves and others and may be a source of stress for teachers.

CONDUCT DISORDER

A conduct disorder is a repetitive and persistent pattern of behaviour in which age-related norms are violated or the rights of others are violated. Young people with conduct disorders may:

+ be aggressive;

+ destroy property;

+ be deceitful.

Young people with conduct disorders violate the rights of others and use intimidation or aggression towards people or animals. They violate others by stealing or destroying their property.

OPPOSITIONAL DEFIANT DISORDER

Young people who have oppositional defiant disorder may:

+ lose their temper or get angry;

+ resent others;

+ argue with those in authority positions;

+ refuse to comply with requests or commands from others;

+ annoy others;

+ blame others;

+ be vindictive towards others.

Oppositional defiant disorder does not include aggression, intimidation or violation against others.

HYPERKINETIC CONDUCT DISORDER

Hyperkinetic conduct disorder is now commonly referred to as attention deficit and hyperactivity disorder (ADHD). Young people in this group may demonstrate the following characteristics:

+ excessive energy or activity;

+ limited attention;

+ lack of perseverance;

+ a tendency to move from activity to activity without completing any task;

+ low self-esteem;

+ delayed motor development;

+ disorganisation.

CASE STUDY

Ryan was in Year 9. He had cognition and learning difficulties. He was underperforming in his literacy skills, but his general knowledge was high. His parents were unemployed and for several years there had been a high degree of parental conflict. Both parents were alcohol dependent and Ryan had witnessed domestic violence in the house. Both parents had developed mental health needs, including depression and anxiety, and his father had self-harmed. Ryan's behaviour had been deteriorating for two years since he started his secondary education. Ryan did not achieve in line with age-related expectations at primary school and on entering secondary school he was placed in the bottom set. He frequently got into fights and he was verbally intimidating to other students and teachers. He had started to truant from school.

CRITICAL QUESTIONS

+ What factors may have resulted in Ryan developing conduct disorders?
+ If you had the role of designated senior lead for mental health, what would you do next to support Ryan?

IDENTIFYING CONDUCT DISORDERS

Signs of conduct disorders include:
+ repetitive and persistent patterns of antisocial, aggressive or defiant behaviour;
+ significant and persistent violations of age-appropriate social expectations.

Aggressive conduct may include:
+ intimidating or bullying others;
+ deliberately physically harming people or animals;
+ using a weapon.

Deceitful behaviour includes:

+ lying;

+ stealing.

Destructive conduct may include intentional destruction of property. Violation of rules may include:

+ truancy;

+ substance abuse;

+ sexual behaviour.

EVIDENCE-BASED APPROACHES TO SUPPORTING YOUNG PEOPLE

Schools need to believe that all young people can improve their behaviour. Demonstrating to young people that you believe in them is one of the most powerful things that you can do to change their behaviour. Additionally, developing effective, respectful and positive relationships with young people is critical in improving their behaviour. Young people respond well when their teachers have high expectations of them. As a teacher, you should communicate high expectations of their behaviour and their academic progress and demonstrate that you have faith in them.

Young people with conduct disorders need to engage in meaningful, relevant and interesting activities. Schools should seek to provide these young people with a practical curriculum which will give them the skills they need for the future. Many young people with conduct disorders will benefit from a curriculum that includes vocational skills development.

It is important to demonstrate empathy; disassociate the behaviour from the person and try to understand that many young people with conduct disorders have experienced multiple forms of adversity and disadvantage in their lives.

Place the young person at the centre of all decision-making processes. This is a key principle of the Special Educational Needs and Disabilities Code of Practice (Department for Education and Department of Health, 2015). Involve them in setting goals and reviewing their own progress, and in planning the curriculum that they will study. Develop positive relationships with their parents and involve parents in decision-making processes. Some parents may need support to understand how their own behaviour may be influencing the behaviour of their child. An effective strategy is to provide parental workshops aimed at helping parents to manage their child's behaviour at home more effectively and teaching parents about the importance of positive relationships and secure attachments at home.

Establishing a whole-school policy of 'no exclusion' is an important step for a school leader to take. Many young people with conduct disorders have been excluded from schools or been involved in 'managed moves'. This is where they are taken off the roll of one school and placed on that of another. The impact of these moves is that they develop a poor sense of self and this can result in a further decline in their behaviour. Demonstrating a whole-school commitment to no exclusion is a real signal that the school is committed to inclusion. One way that schools can achieve this is to develop in-house alternative provision. This helps to maintain a young person's sense of connectivity with the school and their peers.

Evidence of effective intervention supports the use of a curriculum which directly teaches social and emotional skills through small-group intervention programmes (Department for Education, 2016). Young people with conduct disorders may need support in understanding what is meant by socially accepted behaviour and the impact of their behaviour on others. They may need to be taught how to manage their own emotions through a highly structured, systematic intervention programme.

Young people with conduct disorders may benefit from a clear approach to behaviour management that includes the use of rewards and sanctions. They may benefit from a system of rewards and sanctions that is specifically tailored to suit their needs and which they have had the opportunity to shape. However, disproportionate sanctions are not effective and their overuse on a young person might suggest that the use of sanctions is not working. A clear policy on bullying will need to be implemented. The practice of rewards and sanctions is influenced by behaviourism. This is a branch of psychology which emphasises the consequences of behaviour rather than the causes. The work of B F Skinner and the theory of operant conditioning underpin the use of rewards and sanctions.

It is critical that all members of staff in the school understand the specific needs of young people with conduct disorders. Approaches to the management of behaviour are more effective when they are consistently applied. It is important to involve the child in regular goal setting and to provide them with regular informal and formal opportunities to review their own progress.

51

The repertoire of approaches that you adopt to support the child should also draw in elements of a solutions-focused approach. Such an approach does not overtly require the child to revisit their negative behaviour. In contrast, it supports the child in helping them to understand their strengths and thus attempts to build a positive sense of self. Within a solutions-focused approach the child is supported to establish goals that will help to improve the quality of their educational experiences by helping them to recognise that their strengths in one area may be transferable to other areas. There is also some evidence to support the use of nurture groups. A nurture group is a small-group intervention for young people with social and emotional difficulties. Within nurture groups, young people learn in a relaxed, informal physical and emotional environment, which may be representative of a home environment. Within this space the adult focuses on developing social and emotional skills which may be lacking and building a positive sense of self. A solution-focused approach and nurture groups draw on the principles of humanism. This is a branch of psychology which emphasises the importance of self-concept and self-esteem in understanding young people's behaviour. The work of Rogers and Maslow underpin this approach.

SIGNPOSTING FOR FURTHER ADVICE

Parents and young people can access further advice on the following websites:

+ NHS Choices. New guidelines on child antisocial behaviour: www.nhs.uk/news/pregnancy-and-child/new-guidelines-on-child-antisocial-behaviour.

+ Children's Society. Conduct Disorder: www.childrenssociety.org.uk/mental-health-advice-for-children-and-young-people/conduct-disorder.

CRITICAL QUESTIONS

+ Conduct disorders are higher than average in young people of African-Caribbean family origin. What factors might explain this?

+ What factors might exacerbate conduct disorder in young people?

- There has been a 40 per cent increase in permanent exclusions over the past three years.

- 48,000 young people are educated outside of mainstream and special schools during the year.

- In 2015/16, 6,685 pupils were permanently excluded from school. In the same year there were 339,360 fixed-period exclusions.

- Exclusions of young people with special educational needs are disproportionate. In 2015/16, there were 2,990 permanent exclusions and 148,665 fixed-term exclusions of pupils with special educational needs.

- 47 per cent of young people in Alternative Provision are 15–16 years of age.

- 25 per cent of exclusions happen when young people are aged 14, and half of all exclusions happen in Year 9 or above.

(House of Commons Education and Health and Social Care Committees, 2018)

CRITICAL QUESTIONS

+ Why do you think that exclusion rates are so high for young people who have special educational needs?

+ Why do you think that half of all exclusions happen in Year 9 and above?

Some groups of young people are more likely to be educated in Alternative Provision or excluded than others. These include:

+ young people in care;

+ young people in need: those whose home lives have prompted inter-action with social services but who remain in their home environment fare even worse: they are three times more likely to be excluded from their school than other pupils;

+ those with special educational needs and disabilities (SEND): pupils with SEND support are almost seven times more likely to be perman-ently excluded than pupils with no SEND;

+ those in poverty: on average, poorer young people are four times more likely to be excluded than their wealthier peers;

+ boys are more likely to be permanently excluded than girls; for every girl permanently excluded last year, more than three boys were permanently excluded;

+ some ethnicities are disproportionately represented in alternative provision, including Black Caribbean, Irish traveller heritage and Gypsy Roma heritage pupils;

+ pupils who leave primary schools with the lowest skill levels are most likely to be excluded from school.

(Gill et al, 2017)

CRITICAL QUESTIONS

+ Off-rolling is the process by which pupils are removed from the school's register by moving them to alternative provision, to home education or other schools. What might be the effects of this on young people who are moved out of their schools?

+ Why do you think that boys are more likely to develop conduct disorders than girls?

+ Why do you think that looked-after children are at risk of developing conduct disorders?

+ Why do you think that specific ethnic groups are disproportionally represented in alternative provision?

CASE STUDY

A secondary school introduced a peer mentoring scheme. Students in Year 10 were selected to be peer mentors. They were introduced to some simple anger management techniques such as using a punch bag to release excess energy, hitting a wall with a foam bat, going to a calm space, breathing exercises and tearing the anger into pieces. This last technique involved writing or drawing on a piece of paper the things that had upset them and then tearing it up into tiny pieces to 'throw away the anger'. The peer mentors were matched with students in Years 7, 8 and 9 who had been identified as having conduct disorders. The peer mentors introduced their mentees to the anger management strategies through guided one-to-one sessions.

- In January 2017, 186,793 pupils in state-funded mainstream or special schools had social, emotional and mental health as their primary category of special educational need.

- Roughly one in every 50 young people in the general population has social, emotional and mental health needs.

- One in every two pupils in alternative provision has social, emotional and mental health needs.

- 1 per cent of young people in alternative provision get five good GCSEs with English and maths but 99 per cent do not.

(House of Commons Education Committee, 2018)

CRITICAL QUESTIONS

+ The *Special Educational Needs and Disabilities Code of Practice* (Department for Education and Department of Health, 2015) identifies 'social, emotional and mental health needs' as a distinct category of need. Do you agree that mental health needs should sit alongside social and emotional needs?

+ Why do you think that so few young people in alternative provision gain good GCSE results?

Research has found that racist stereotypes have been shown to unconsciously bias teachers' perceptions of behaviour and pupils' personalities, particularly with black students (Okonofua and Eberhardt, 2015). Research shows that although black young people begin school with similar attainment to their peers, on average they fall behind drastically through secondary school (Shaw et al, 2016).

55

Researchers have also found that a two-way relationship exists between child and adolescent mental illness and exclusion from school (Parker et al, 2016). Thus, young people with mental health needs are more likely to be excluded and exclusion can also result in mental health needs.

SUMMARY

This chapter has outlined some of the reasons why young people develop conduct disorders and introduced you to some strategies that you can use to support students to improve their behaviour. While it may not be your intention to teach in alternative provision, a short experiential placement in alternative provision will be extremely beneficial to your development as a teacher. It is here that you will meet some of the most marginalised young people who have multiple complex needs. It is in alternative provision that you will meet hard-working, dedicated and resilient teachers and support staff who are committed to raising the aspirations of these marginalised young people. The important point to remember is that when young people abuse you it is rarely a personal attack at you. Often, it is an attempt to communicate an unmet need. Young people will often hurt those who care for them the most. Your duty as a teacher is to help them to realise that they can change their behaviour and that their life chances do not have to be determined by their previous experiences. You are the person who can change their mindset. You are the one who can build their self-esteem and confidence. You are the one who can raise their aspirations and you are the person who can convince them that they can improve. This is the reason why you came into teaching in the first place. Never lose sight of that.

CHECKLIST

This chapter has addressed:

✓ the importance of demonstrating to young people that you believe in them;

✓ the importance of not giving up on any student;

✓ the role of the family, school and individual factors in contributing to conduct disorders;

✓ the groups of young people who are more likely to end up in alternative provision.

FURTHER READING

Delaney, M (2008) *Teaching the Unteachable: Practical Ideas to Give Teachers Hope and Help When Behaviour Management Strategies Fail: What Teachers Can Do When All Else Fails*. Belper: Worth Publishing.

Delaney, M (2017) *Attachment for Teachers: The Essential Handbook for Trainee Teachers and NQTs*. Belper: Worth Publishing.

✚ CHAPTER 4

IDENTIFYING AND SUPPORTING YOUNG PEOPLE WHO SELF-HARM

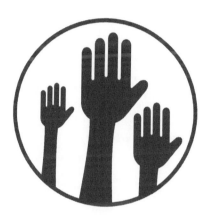

PROFESSIONAL LINKS

This chapter addresses the following:

- Schools have a statutory responsibility to keep young people safe. Full information about the safeguarding duty can be found in the Department for Education (2016) statutory guidance *Keeping Children Safe in Education: Statutory Guidance for Schools and Colleges.*

- This duty extends to all teachers through the *Teachers' Standards* (2011).

CHAPTER OBJECTIVES

By the end of this chapter you will understand:

+ why young people self-harm;

+ types of self-harm;

+ how to support young people who self-harm.

INTRODUCTION

It is extremely concerning when young people self-harm because of the risks that are associated with it. It is still the case that self-harm is stigmatised. Some adults cannot understand why young people inflict harm on themselves and consequently they cast negative judgement on victims of self-harm. There are many myths relating to self-harm, which need to be explicitly stated. These are identified below.

+ Self-harm is usually not a manipulative act.

+ It is usually not a form of attention seeking, as many young people try to hide the evidence of the self-harm.

+ It is usually not a failed suicide attempt; people who self-harm are not usually suicidal.

+ It is usually not carried out for pleasure.

+ It is not an indication of a personality disorder.

+ The seriousness of the injury is not related to the seriousness of the problem.

+ It is not carried out because victims like pain; it is often a way of coping.

+ Self-harm is not a young person's issue; people of all ages self-harm.

+ It is not easy to stop self-harming.

+ The problems do not go away if the self-harm stops.

This chapter addresses some of the reasons why young people self-harm, the types of self-harm and ways in which schools can support young people who self-harm.

FACTORS THAT RESULT IN SELF-HARM

Self-harm occurs when someone hurts or harms their body. Often, self-harm is understood to be an act that causes immediate physical damage to the body. However, many people harm their bodies in ways that are not usually considered forms of self-harm. Examples include excessive eating, excessive drinking, drug abuse and smoking.

CRITICAL QUESTIONS

+ Is self-harm a choice?

+ Is it a deliberate act?

+ Do you consider excessive eating, excessive drinking, drug abuse and smoking to be forms of self-harm? Explain your views.

The experience of physical and emotional changes that occur during adolescence, particularly during puberty, can lead to self-harm. If there is evidence of self-harm or attempted suicide in the family or if a friend has engaged in self-harm this can increase the risk of a young person self-harming. Adverse family circumstances, dysfunctional relationships, domestic violence, poverty, parental criminality and being taken into care can also result in self-harm. Young people who self-harm may have experienced physical, emotional or sexual abuse during childhood. Self-harm is more common among young people who suffer from mental health disorders. These factors can result in anxiety and depression, which can subsequently result in self-harm.

Some young people discover that the experience of pain changes their mood. This may then become habit forming. Cutting the skin releases endorphins, which produce brief feelings of calm, and serotonin, which lifts the mood.

Self-harm often starts with other mental health conditions such as depression or anxiety. Understanding why someone is depressed or anxious can help to get to the root of the problem. If the causes can be addressed, this can alleviate or eradicate the depression or anxiety which are causing the self-harm. However, it is important to emphasise that self-harm can occur with no previous history of mental health problems and people do it for a range of reasons. These include:

+ to reduce tension;

+ to manage extreme emotional upset;

+ to distract them from emotional pain;

+ to express hurt, anger or frustration;

+ to regain a sense of control;

+ to punish themselves;

+ to communicate with others that they need help;

+ to identify with a peer group;

+ to express something that is difficult to put into words;

+ to turn invisible thoughts or feelings into something visible;

+ to change emotional pain into physical pain;

+ to escape traumatic memories;

+ to have something in their life that they can rely on;

+ to stop feeling numb, disconnected or dissociated;

+ to create a reason to physically care for themselves;

+ to express suicidal feelings and thoughts without taking their own life.

(Mind: www.mind.org.uk).

Over time, self-harming can become a habit that is hard to stop. At its most extreme, self-harm can be a suicide attempt. However, this is usually not the case. There may be no single cause of self-harm and multiple factors intersect which causes an individual to cause harm to their body.

CRITICAL QUESTIONS

+ What school factors may result in self-harm?

+ What psychological factors may result in self-harm?

+ What social factors may result in self-harm?

Self-harm can be categorised as follows.

+ Individual factors: for example, low self-esteem; identity issues.

+ Family factors: for example, parental conflict; poor family relationships; family history of self-harm; abuse and neglect.

+ Social factors: for example, peer rejection; bullying or negative peer influences.

TYPES OF SELF-HARM

Ways of self-harming can include:

+ *cutting;*

+ *poisoning;*

+ *over- or under-eating;*

+ *biting;*

+ *picking or scratching at the skin;*

+ *burning the skin with cigarettes, aerosols and scalding;*

+ *inserting objects into the body;*

+ *hitting oneself or walls;*

+ *overdosing;*

+ *exercising excessively;*

+ *pulling the hair;*

+ *getting into fights where getting hurt is inevitable.*

(Mind: www.mind.org.uk).

IDENTIFYING SELF-HARM

Young people may be reluctant to disclose their self-harming because they may not believe it will be treated in confidence. If the young person's safety and welfare is at risk then adults in school are legally required to refer them to specialist services. However, some forms of self-harm do not immediately place a young person at risk and therefore not all young people need to be referred to specialist services.

After self-harming, a young person may experience a sense of shame and embarrassment at their actions. They may hide the visible signs of self-harm. Some may feel ashamed, not only of the self-harm itself, but also of the reasons why they self-harmed. Many young people experience a sense of shame at their own actions but also recognise that other people may also respond negatively to their actions. Thus, the sense of shame is heightened. They may become secretive and cover up their injuries. It is important for all adults working in school to suspend judgement and to create a climate of trust.

Warning signs may include:

+ unexplained burns, cuts, scars, or other clusters of similar markings on the skin;

+ arms, hands and forearms opposite the dominant hand are common areas for self-harm, although self-harm can take place on other parts of the body;

+ inappropriate dress for the season, such as consistently wearing long sleeves or trousers in the summer;

+ constant use of wrist bands or other coverings;

+ unwillingness to participate in events or activities that require less clothing;

+ frequently wearing bandages;

+ increased signs of depression or anxiety.

Young people often reach a point when they want to stop self-harming for a range of reasons. These include:

+ *starting to 'grow out' of it – it begins to feel like an immature way to deal with life problems;*

+ *wanting to find other, more positive, ways of coping and to improve their overall mental health;*

+ *wanting to take care of their physical health;*

+ *feeling the shame and/or embarrassment of their actions;*

+ *the secrecy is becoming too overwhelming and uncomfortable;*

+ *wishing to avoid negative reactions from others;*

+ *disliking the physical scars self-harm leaves behind;*

+ *recognising the pain it causes to their friends and families;*

+ *realising that it is no longer working or helping them to cope.*

(Healthy Young Minds: http://healthyyoungmindspennine.nhs.uk)

- 60 per cent of teachers say that they do not feel able to talk about self-harm.

- Two-thirds of teachers thought that they would say the wrong thing if someone turned to them for help with self-harm.

- 80 per cent of teachers said they wanted practical advice on how to help.

(Anna Freud National Centre for Children and Families: www.annafreud.org)

EVIDENCE-BASED APPROACHES TO SUPPORT YOUNG PEOPLE

This section covers approaches that schools can adopt to support young people who self-harm.

MANAGING ADULT REACTIONS

Adult reactions (including those of teachers and other staff in school) to self-harming can vary. They include sadness, alarm, panic, anxiety and shock. Adults may be scared, distressed, upset, repulsed, bewildered and frustrated.

Adults should try to suspend negative reactions because the young person may already be experiencing a sense of shame or guilt. It is important to focus on how you can help the young person rather than how you feel about what they have done.

REDUCING STIGMA

Self-harm is surrounded with prejudice and stigma. Schools play a critical role in breaking down the stigma by talking openly about self-harm. The more that we cover something up by 'sweeping it under the carpet', the more likely stigma will develop. By talking with young people and parents about self-harm schools can help to tackle the myths around self-harm.

CRITICAL QUESTIONS

Reflect on the following questions.

+ What do you know about emotional wellbeing?

+ How well do you understand self-harm?

+ What can you do to tackle stigma in your school and community?

+ How can you involve young people more in discussions about self-harm?

+ How can you involve young people in a campaign to tackle stigma or support young people to run their own campaign?

MANAGING A DISCLOSURE

The following advice is useful for managing disclosures of self-harm.

+ Do not panic! It is important to talk about the issue and acknowledge how brave the young person is for speaking to you.

+ Listen to the young person: listen to them and try not to interrupt; suspend judgement.

+ Do not tell them to 'just stop doing it': they are doing it as a coping mechanism, not as a form of manipulating other people. It is not easy for them to stop doing it. The underlying causes need to be addressed first.

+ Make a plan: involve the young person in developing a plan of 'ways forward'. Provide them with ownership so that they are not being told what to do. Advise them of the school-based support that is available and offer to take them to the school counsellor or pastoral department.

+ If someone is actively suicidal, stay calm and make sure that they are safe with someone so that you can go and seek advice from the designated safeguarding lead; if they have already taken an overdose then you will need to call an ambulance immediately. Do not try to drive the young person to the hospital yourself.

+ Thank the young person for speaking to you and explain to them what will happen next. Explain who you will need to share the information with and why it needs to be shared; explain what will happen next.

+ Document the discussion immediately after it has taken place. Keep the record factual and do not add your own interpretations.

+ Speak to the designated safeguarding lead about the next steps and whether a referral is required; the safeguarding lead will coordinate it from this point forward.

+ Keep the young person informed about what is happening and keep 'checking in' on them.

PEER SUPPORT

Friends can play a significant role in helping people get the support they need. Many schools train peer mentors or student ambassadors to become 'peer listeners'. Young people may prefer to speak to other young people rather than an adult in school or a family member. The peer mentors will need training in:

+ how to listen without interruption;

+ how to suspend judgement;

+ confidentiality and referral to a member of staff in school;

+ how to put the young person in control by asking them what support they need;

+ developing empathy.

A range of models of peer support exists, including informal drop-in sessions and 'buddy' systems. Schools will need to consider what criteria will be applied for selecting peer mentors and a selection process will need to be designed.

SCHOOL NURSE

The school nurse can play a critical role in supporting young people who self-harm. The nurse can provide health advice, particularly in relation to managing stress, anxiety and depression. These factors might result in self-harm. Additionally, the school nurse can contribute to delivering the mental health curriculum and they can advise school staff on how to manage cases of self-harm.

SPEAKING TO A DOCTOR

The young person might need to be signposted to a doctor if they require medical advice. Doctors will usually not share the information with parents but there are instances when they may be required to do this.

RELAXATION TECHNIQUES

Relaxation techniques can help to reduce stress, which may be an under-lying cause of self-harm. Examples of relaxation techniques include:

+ listening to calm music;

+ deep breathing;

+ visualisation techniques with eyes closed;

+ intensely focusing on an object;

+ peer massage.

MINDFULNESS

Mindfulness is an approach which supports people to enjoy 'being within the moment'. The activity encourages the use of the senses to enjoy an experience. Often, we do not enjoy experiences because we are rushing and thinking more about what we need to do next. This can result in limiting pleasure and happiness, which improve mental health. Mindfulness focuses the attention away from what has happened in the past and what is likely to happen in the future. Negative experiences from the past and negative thoughts about the future can result in self-harm. Mindfulness takes the attention away from these experiences and focuses the mind on enjoying what is happening in the present. Mindfulness activities can take a variety of forms. An example would be mindful eating with an item of food. The activity would focus attention on what the food looks like, what it feels like and what it smells like, before the food is placed in the mouth. When the food is placed in the mouth, it would be placed on the tongue before being chewed. The eating of the food would be completed slowly rather than quickly, and the focus would be on what the food tastes like. Mindfulness can be a useful strategy for young people to try at home when they are feeling stressed, depressed or anxious.

CRITICAL QUESTIONS

+ How might you structure a mindful walking activity with young people?

+ How might you build mindfulness into the curriculum?

+ To what extent might the busy nature of school life contribute to poor mental health?

PHYSICAL ACTIVITY

Physical activity improves mental health. If the self-harm has been caused because the young person has underlying mental health needs, such as depression, physical activity can be an effective tool for helping people to feel better.

SIGNPOSTING FOR FURTHER ADVICE

Unless a child or young person's self-harming poses a safeguarding concern, you must obtain their consent to share information about them. When information is shared, young people need to be informed about:

+ who the information is shared with;

+ what information will be shared;

+ why the information is being shared.

Young people should be signposted to the school nurse, counsellor or pastoral team for support. Additionally, the following organisations can provide confidential advice and information to young people who self-harm:

+ selfharmUK: www.selfharm.co.uk
+ Childline: www.childline.org.uk
+ the Samaritans: www.samaritans.org.uk
+ Youth Access: www.youthaccess.co.uk
+ Youth 2 Youth: www.youth2youth.co.uk
+ Mind: www.mind.org.uk
+ Harmless: www.harmless.org.uk
+ National Self-Harm Network: www.nshn.co.uk
+ YoungMinds: https://youngminds.org.uk

SPEAKING TO THE PARENTS

It is important to stress that many young people who self-harm will not want their parents to know that they are self-harming. They may not want to worry their parents or they may be self-harming because of their parents. However, in most instances the information will need to be shared with parents and carers and with other organisations. The young person needs to be informed why this is necessary, what information will be shared and what will happen next. If the self-harm has been caused by parental abuse and neglect, then the school safeguarding policy should be followed. There may be situations where informing the young person's parents might place them in more danger. In these situations, it is not appropriate to inform the parents.

One in 12 children in the UK deliberately self-harms.

25,000 young people are sent to accident and emergency departments in hospital every year because of their injuries from self-harming.

(YoungMinds: https://youngminds.org.uk)

Research (Fox and Hawton, 2004) has shown that the experiences most closely linked to self-harm in young people are:

+ mental health problems (including hopelessness and depression);

+ family issues (such as parental criminality and/or family poverty);

+ disrupted upbringing (being in local authority care, parental marital problems, separation or divorce);

+ being abused;

+ continuing family relationship problems.

The National Institute for Health and Care Excellence (2004) has indicated that those who have self-harmed are 100 times more likely than the general population to die by suicide in the following year. The risk increases for those who self-harm repeatedly. Self-harm is therefore a strong risk factor for suicide.

CASE STUDY

A secondary school introduced some strategies for managing feelings for young people who were self-harming. The strategies included:

+ clenching an ice cube in the hand until it melts;

+ snapping an elastic band against the wrist;

+ drawing on the skin with a red pen or red paint instead of cutting;

+ sports or physical exercise;

+ using a punchbag;

+ hitting a pillow or other soft object;

+ listening to or creating loud music.

The students used these strategies instead of self-harming and there was a reduction in the number of incidents.

- There has been a 68 per cent rise in rates of self-harm among girls aged 13–16 since 2011.
- In the UK between 2010 and 2015, suicide rates among 15–19 year-olds rose from 3.2 to 5.4 per 100,000.

(Morgan et al, 2017)

CRITICAL QUESTIONS

+ Why do you think that girls are more likely to self-harm than boys?

+ Why do you think there is a correlation between self-harm and suicide?

Some research suggests that self-harm is more common in some youth subcultures. This may be because young people emulate cultural icons or peers who self-harm. Alternatively, the link between self-harm and youth subcultures could be explained because those with a particular propensity to self-harm are attracted to the subculture.

(Grant and Potenza, 2007, p 372)

CASE STUDY

A secondary school put on a workshop for parents on self-harm. The workshop addressed:

+ what self-harm is;

+ the signs of self-harm;

+ ways in which parents can support their child who is self-harming;

+ sources of support online and in the community.

In the same school, a group of young people who had previously self-harmed organised a student-led conference on self-harm for all Year 7 students. The conference provided young people with a range of authentic voices on self-harm. A series of interactive workshops were led by young people on the theme of self-harm.

SUMMARY

This chapter has outlined many of the myths that surround self-harm. It has emphasised how stigma can prevent young people from speaking about self-harm and it has stressed the need for adults to suspend judgement. Young people do not self-harm because they are self-centred or attention seeking. They self-harm because it is a way of coping with adverse experiences. They experience feelings of guilt and shame and they blame themselves. It is important that young people know that it is not their fault but that their actions are a response to the adverse experiences that have affected them. Unless self-harm is de-stigmatised, young people will continue to be secretive about it by not speaking about it and hiding the evidence. Schools play a critical role in de-stigmatising self-harm by opening up the conversation.

CHECKLIST

This chapter has addressed:

✓ the factors that can result in self-harm;

✓ the signs of self-harm;

✓ ways in which you can support young people who self-harm.

FURTHER READING

Fitzpatrick, C (2012) *A Short Introduction to Understanding and Supporting Children and Young People Who Self-harm*. London: Jessica Kingsley.

McDougall, T, Armstrong, M and Trainor, G (2010) *Helping Children and Young People who Self-harm: An Introduction to Self-harming and Suicidal Behaviours for Health Professionals*. London: Routledge.

✚ CHAPTER 5

IDENTIFYING AND SUPPORTING SPECIFIC AT-RISK GROUPS

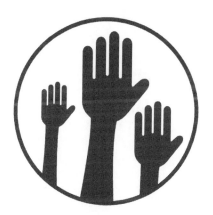

PROFESSIONAL LINKS

This chapter addresses the following:

- The Departments for Education and Health document *Transforming Children and Young People's Mental Health Provision: A Green Paper* (2017), including proposals from the government about early intervention and prevention for individuals in at-risk groups.

- The NHS 'Mental Health Workforce Strategy' (2017).

- The Child and Social Work Act (2017).

CHAPTER OBJECTIVES

By the end of this chapter you will understand:

+ how to help and support the following at-risk groups of young people:
  - care leavers;
  - those who experience domestic abuse;
  - young people involved in gang culture;
  - refugees and asylum seekers.

INTRODUCTION

This chapter provides you with an introduction to the knowledge and skills needed to help some of the student groups who are at a significantly higher risk of suffering from mental health issues. If you are already in a position where you work with children and young people then you will, we hope, already be making a huge positive difference to them by being a calm and stable figure in their lives. Some of the knowledge and ideas proposed in this chapter will help you to do this even more, by further developing the skills needed to help these groups of young people to achieve success through helping protect their mental health as they develop into young adults under your care and provision.

The NHS has published its Mental Health Workforce Strategy (2017), in which it promised to improve the quality and provision of mental health care by recruiting and training an additional 2000 child and adolescent mental health services staff by 2020/21. This strategy is to try and improve access to services for 70,000 children and young people over the next few years. However, until these services are 'up and running' we hope this chapter will provide some basic knowledge about ideas for good practice that can be implemented to bring about positive change for those children and young people who need it the most at this time.

HELPING MEET THE MENTAL HEALTH NEEDS OF CARE LEAVERS

A 'child in care' often refers to a child living with foster parents, or one at home with their parents but under close supervision from social services, a child living in residential settings such as a secure unit. The child may have been placed in care by parents struggling to cope or, often, when children's services have been forced to intervene because there is a high risk of harm.

Research has been undertaken to look at how well those in care transition out of the care system to live independent lives. The research highlighted alarming results. The charity Barnardo's found that of 274 care leavers, 125 had mental health needs and, of those individuals, only 35 per cent were receiving the specialist support they needed from mental health services. Furthermore, one in four care leavers had experienced a mental health crisis since leaving care (Smith, 2017). This section begins by outlining the provision that local authorities are legally bound to provide care leavers to protect their mental and physical health and wellbeing. This dissection describes ways in which you can help care leavers during this time too.

The research from Barnardo's (Smith, 2017) presents an alarming trend in the number of care leavers failing to receive appropriate health care when they need it. It is clear that care leavers face complex psychological difficulties. For many young people, the transition between being a child who is wholly cared and provided for to being an independent adult is a smoother transition where responsibility shifts from carer to young person gently over time. Care leavers are often faced with the opposite situation, with many overlapping changes that can impact on their living situation all at once. Recent changes to Section 3 of the Children and Social Work Act 2017 mean that local authorities now have responsibility to provide what is called a 'personal advisor' to all care leavers up to the age of 25 years. Local authorities have to publish what is called a 'local offer' which sets out the care leaver's legal entitlements and any additional support they will provide, and they must apply seven principles set out by parliament, which include the following:

+ *to act in the best interests, and promote the physical and mental health and well-being, of those children and young people;*

+ *to encourage those children and young people to express their views, wishes and feelings;*

+ *to take into account the views, wishes and feelings of those children and young people;*

+ *to help those children and young people gain access to, and make the best use of, services provided by the local authority and its relevant partners;*

+ to promote high aspirations, and seek to secure the best outcomes, for those children and young people;

+ for those children and young people to be safe, and for stability in their home lives, relationships and education or work;

+ to prepare those children and young people for adulthood and independent living.

(Children and Social Work Act, 2017)

The ultimate aim that the current government hopes to achieve from the above seven principles is that care leavers are well supported to live successful and independent lives. The aim of these proposed plans is that support will taper off over time, as is the case with general parenting of young people not in care. For care leavers aged 16–17 years, the local authority must provide accommodation for them, alongside a personal adviser for support. For those aged 18–20 years, the local authority must maintain a good level of communication with them to ensure they are well supported. For those aged 21–25 years, the local authority must assess their needs and develop and review a pathway plan when the individual in question requests support. This new legislation was implemented to ensure that, in theory, no young care leaver should be left isolated or to fend for themselves. While this book is aimed at helping to support you in your work with young people aged 11–18 years, it is important you know the legal framework in which local authorities are legally bound to work once the young person is between the ages of 18 and 25 years.

Children's early experiences can profoundly affect their development and the chances of them living successful and healthy lives. Because of difficult experiences before and during care means that looked-after children are always at higher risk of mental health issues than their peers. While still at school, those who are in the care system regularly have a highly disruptive experience in the education system through regularly having to move to a new house, change schools or be taken out of school for meetings. To best support these children and young people, they need those working close to them to develop strong, trusting and stable relationships. Those involved in caring for them and looking after them while they are at school need high-quality training and support to help meet their mental needs.

Children and young people often enter care because they have been abused or neglected, which can result in them having a range of complicated emotional and mental health needs. These needs can increase their vulnerable status and make them more susceptible to abuse. To attempt to protect the mental health needs of those in care and those leaving care, the NSPCC (2018) has outlined six guidelines which can help transform improvements in the provision offered to these children and young people:

+ ensure that they are given an opportunity to have their voices heard;

+ strengthen the social care workforce and improve practice;

+ promote their right to advocacy so they can be supported to express their views;

+ improve emotional support offered to these children and young people;

+ provide more intense support when transitioning into and out of care;

+ improve the public understanding of the care system.

While you may feel that a number of the above points are issues beyond your control, consider whether there are any you could put into practice in your workplace to help improve mental health provision for the children that you work with.

CRITICAL QUESTIONS

+ How can you create an environment which better lends itself to providing more opportunities to listen to the voices of the children in care or recent care leavers who you work closely with?

+ How can you help promote their right to advocacy in your work with children?

+ Are there any areas in which you think you could provide better emotional support?

+ As a teacher, how can you contribute to helping improve the public understanding of the care system?

HELPING THOSE WHO EXPERIENCE DOMESTIC ABUSE

The Royal College of Psychiatrists (2018) defines 'domestic abuse' as encompassing a specific incident or a series of incidents, of controlling and threatening behaviour, violence or abuse. This can include physical (for example, throwing objects), as well as sexual and emotional abuse (including verbal threats and controlling behaviour). Honour-based violence and forced marriages are also types of domestic abuse. As technology continues to advance, it is becoming more common for domestic abuse to happen on mobile phones, on social networking sites and the internet. It no longer only has to take place in the home. It is thought that, in adult relationships where there is domestic violence and abuse, children and young people witness about 75 per cent of the abusive incidents and about 50 per cent of the children in these families have themselves been badly hit or beaten (Royal College of Psychiatrists, 2018). A child can be affected by domestic violence and abuse even when still in the womb.

Regular domestic abuse in the home can result in children and young people suffering from anxiety. It may show itself in physiological symptoms such as constant stomach aches or headaches, or behaviours such as wetting the bed at an older than expected age. The child may also behave immaturely. Children and young people may express their distress by behaving more aggressively and defiantly, and may copy the behaviour they see within the family home. Many will drift into alcohol and drug abuse, attempting to block the disturbing memories they may have or to numb themselves to the realities of their home lives. Many children and young people will blame it on themselves. This can increase the likelihood of mental health issues such as eating disorders, the regular desire to self-harm or having suicidal feelings. They are also more likely to choose an abusive partner who treats them in an equally derogatory manner. They may experience post-traumatic stress disorder (PTSD) and may suffer from flash-backs or become very jumpy. Those children who experience domestic abuse at home typically have lower educational outcomes than their peers (Royal College of Psychiatrists, 2018), perhaps as a result of difficult or terrifying memories or of being so worried about an abused parent they may become a school-refuser (a child who refuses to attend school regularly).

To try to protect the mental health of any children or young people who are experiencing these symptoms, an important point to remember and reinforce from the outset is that these issues at home do not have to be kept secret and can be discussed. Appearances can be very deceptive when it comes to domestic abuse, so it is important you do not simply take children's responses as fact and you delve deeper if you are concerned that there may be an issue underneath the surface.

In the first instance, your school's or centre's safeguarding policy must be followed and the relevant safeguarding officer must be made aware and appropriate steps must be taken. Children and young people can be signposted to professional services such as individual or group treatments for children suffering from particular mental health disorders, such as stress, anxiety and PTSD. There are a number of healthcare professionals, including doctors, nurses, health visitors, talk therapists and qualified counsellors, who can help them to heal over time.

Children can often be in denial about what they have seen or experienced as for them it is 'normal' and they know little else. Having just one strong relationship with a trustworthy adult can make a huge difference in their lives as they will feel more open to discussing the problems, which can lead to the child being helped more quickly and can result in less of a negative long-term impact on the child. While you may feel helpless, remember that you could be that one person who is a constant source of peace, continuity and reliability for them; just by being there for them and talking to them you have the power to make a huge difference in their lives.

- Around one in five children has been exposed to domestic abuse.
- Domestic abuse is a factor in over half of serious case reviews.
- One-third of children witnessing domestic violence have also experienced another form of abuse.

(NSPCC, www.nspcc.org.uk)

Abuse and neglect by parents or guardians was found to be associated with children and young people's poorer emotional wellbeing, including current thoughts about self-harm and suicidal ideation. Witnessing domestic violence was also related to poorer emotional wellbeing. Experiencing physical violence from a parent or guardian and witnessing domestic violence were also associated with higher levels of delinquent behaviour.

(Radford et al, 2011)

HELPING THOSE INVOLVED IN GANG-AFFILIATED CULTURE

There are many reasons why young people feel that they should join a gang. For some this varies from boredom to the need for more excitement, thrill and adrenaline in their lives. For other young people who regularly suffer from insecure feelings or those who are regularly victimised, they may like the status or powerful feelings that being in a gang can provide them. For many children and young people it can give them a sense of belonging for the first time in their lives. Public Health England (2015) released a report entitled *The Mental Health Needs of Gang-Affiliated Young People*. This report includes an outline of the shared risk factors for poor mental health and gang affiliation, which include:

+ attachment insecurity and poor care-giver bonds;

+ child abuse and neglect;

+ non-intact family;

+ a parent who suffered from postnatal depression;

+ a history of mental illness in families.

There is a clear link between poor mental health and young people affiliated with gangs, but the report also highlights how they face serious adversity and often have multiple physical and social needs. To best support their mental health needs, these young people need signposting and access to a range of evidence-based and non-stigmatising interventions to help move them away from gang culture and heal any mental and physical health problems they may be suffering. There are often 'local care pathways', set up by local councils to help to provide specialist support for those young people needing professional help. There is a lack of research on how successful these interventions are for young people, especially for young women.

Conduct disorder is most common in young people in gang-affiliated culture. This is a mental health disorder characterised by a major disregard for and aggression towards others, and any behaviours which result in a difference in power, such as aggression or coercion, are gratifying to the individual (Child Mind Institute, 2018). Recommended interventions for this condition include cognitive behavioural therapy (CBT) through qualified counsellors and therapists. When working with young people suffering from conduct disorder, these sessions may cover social and cognitive skills training, moral reasoning and anger management. There are different versions of CBT for children suffering with mental health issues and involved in gang-affiliated culture; for example, aggression replacement training is a cognitive behavioural intervention directly aimed at helping young people who show regular aggressive and violent behaviour. This is just one example of many of the different types of CBT-related programmes that should be available to young people affiliated with gangs in your local area.

These young people may also have been exposed to traumatic events. Trauma-focused CBT (known in short as 'TF-CBT') focuses on managing the anxiety and modifying maladaptive (irrational) thoughts related to the traumatic experience to which the young person has been exposed. There are other therapeutic approaches that Public Health England (2015) recommends including eye movement desensitisation and processing. This is a form of psychotherapy that uses two attention exercises which help to disrupt stored memories of trauma.

With many issues stemming from poor family relationships at home, there are some family-focused therapies, such as functional family therapy and multisystemic therapy (for those at high risk of being placed in care or custody from repeat offending and/or poor behaviour). There are worthwhile programmes to signpost parents and families who are struggling to cope. Mentoring programmes have been proven to be really effective in helping young people, particularly in helping provide a non-family adult role model. Mentors with personal gang culture experience are particularly effective. An effective mentoring programme worth looking at for inspiration and ideas is London's 'SOS Project' (St Giles Trust, 2018), which provides one-to-one support to those involved in gangs across London's most deprived areas.

To effectively help in lessening the risk of poor mental health leading to gang-affiliated culture, and to help those who are already affiliated, there needs to be good collaborative work and connections between different services. We hope that this section of the book has provided an outline of some of the options you should have available in your area to help you in your work with young people struggling with gang culture and/or the associated mental health risks.

CASE STUDY

Amy had felt slightly ignored at home recently. Her parents had decided to divorce and were constantly shouting and arguing about money.

Home was no longer a relaxing place, so Amy hung out on the streets more. She felt a bit lonely as she did not have that many friends at school and she felt that no boys were ever interested in her. She felt completely invisible and unimportant. She was also really bored with nothing to do outside of school time. Her parents were so busy with work and arguing that they had got into the habit of forgetting to text her when she was out to see if she was okay and she had no specific time she had to return home by. So Amy felt free but also pretty ignored at the same time and she felt nobody cared about her.

She joined a gang out of sheer boredom, dying to be noticed and have some fun and adrenaline in her 'boring' life again. Finally she felt like people were interested in her and that she belonged! Over time, however, some of the things the other gang members were doing began to really bother her. They were shouting out offensive things to other strangers walking by and they regularly stole stuff. She felt pressured to join in with these activities and so she did. Amy knew this kind of behaviour was against the values she had been brought up with and she was also in constant fear of her parents finding out, but she could not escape gang life. She was approached in school by her form tutor who had heard about the lifestyle Amy had drifted into. She agreed to attend an outside-school mentoring programme run by a local charity.

The programme focused on mentoring her through emotional and behavioural change. Amy could not believe that another adult, who was not a family member, would take time out on a voluntary basis to help her. The programme helped Amy to create a plan to escape out of the gang. Since she left the gang, a number of its members are now in prison for knife crimes. Amy is so glad she escaped in time before things got that bad, and she was grateful for the mentoring programme that helped her create a 'way out'. She has now made a new group of friends through the charity who she hangs out with in her free time, and she is significantly happier and more at peace with herself and her family situation.

CRITICAL QUESTIONS

+ What signs of gang association might you be able to spot in a young person?

+ What issues might stop a young person seeking help and how could this be overcome?

HELPING REFUGEES AND ASYLUM SEEKERS

Young people who are new to the United Kingdom may arrive as refugees or asylum seekers. Some of them may have experienced war and conflict in their home countries. They may have witnessed tragic events, including the loss of their homes and possessions. Some may have witnessed and/or experienced the death or torture of family members, friends and people from their communities. These negative experiences can have a significant and detrimental effect on their mental health and some will have PTSD.

The migration from their home countries to the United Kingdom may have been traumatic. They may have been separated from members of their family. They may have spent long periods of time travelling, followed by several months living in camps. These young people are uncertain of what their future will look like. They have no guarantees of arriving safely, remaining with their families and finding a home. This can lead to stress, anxiety and depression.

When they arrive in a new country they must settle in a new community. They may not know anyone in that community apart from the people they have arrived with. They may not speak the language. The adults who are responsible for them must try to find work so that they can provide for their families. They may experience harassment and discrimination in their new communities from people who resent them being there. Young people who are refugees and asylum seekers may be anxious about family members who are left behind in their home communities. They may be worried about their safety.

Then they must attend a new school. It is likely that they may not know anyone in the school. The systems, rules and routines are unfamiliar to them. The curriculum is different from the curriculum they studied back at home and the teachers do not know them at first.

These young people experience complex and multiple transitions all within the same period. Transitions are difficult for all young people. Changing class, changing school and moving home can result in stress, anxiety and depression for all young people. However, for refugees and asylum seekers, transitioning to a new country, to a new language and to a completely new community, having fled from war, disaster and threat can result in persistent mental health needs. These young people may face an uncertain future. Until they gain asylum, there is no guarantee that they will be allowed to stay in their new country. They may live with the constant fear that they will have to return home to a country that is unstable.

While schools cannot remove these negative experiences, there is a great deal that schools can do to ensure that young people who are refugees and asylum seekers have a smooth transition to their new school.

School leaders should ensure that there is a positive culture in the school which promotes respect, kindness, care, inclusion and acceptance. This will help young people who are refugees and asylum seekers to experience a sense of belonging. Experiencing a sense of belonging and connectedness to the school is essential to the development of positive mental health.

School leaders should meet with the young person before they formally start at the school to welcome them into the school community. It is important to explain the school routines and to provide a tour of the school so that they are familiar with the layout of the building. They will need to be issued a timetable in advance. They will need to know which classrooms to go to and the location of any storage facilities. Bilingual support may be essential at this point if the young person is new to English.

Schools may wish to consider providing the young person with a peer buddy. This is someone who can meet with them at the start of the day and at key times such as break times and lunch times to provide them with practical and emotional support. If the young person speaks some English, this will greatly support this process. If they do not speak English, then it is still helpful to see a familiar face each day. If bilingual support is available, and it may not be, this will be useful to facilitate communication between the buddy and the young person.

Teachers should provide the young person with a seat in class so that they know where to sit. Teachers might find it useful to prepare the class before they arrive by discussing ways in which they can help the new student. In secondary schools it might be appropriate for the form teacher to do this. During the first few weeks, a named member of staff should be given responsibility to 'check-in' regularly with the student. This might be a pastoral worker who is able to offer emotional support. This person may also wish to check-in on a weekly basis with the family so that lines of communication between home and school are clear.

The young person may need support during unstructured time such as during breaks, lunch times and free periods. A peer buddying system could be implemented during these times so that the young person is not left alone.

Teachers should provide opportunities during lessons for group work. This will give the young person an opportunity to develop social connections. It will also give them an opportunity to start to learn the language. Young people master new languages quickly when they are immersed in a social and communicative environment. Teachers should establish positive relationships with the young person so that they feel safe. High-quality teacher–student relationships help the young person to form an attachment with their teachers. Attachment is not synonymous with dependency. Use of praise in the classroom will help to develop a positive sense of self in the young person.

Teachers need to provide high-quality inclusive teaching. Young people who are refugees and asylum seekers do not need anything different to this. High-quality inclusive teaching benefits all young people. Teachers should:

+ provide clear, concise explanations of subject content;

+ support explanations with visual cues;

+ support explanations with modelling so that new learning is demonstrated as well as being verbally explained;

+ use a multisensory approach which draws on all sensory channels as a vehicle for promoting learning;

+ consider whether the use of writing frames and graphic organisers will be beneficial;

+ provide pre-teaching where this will aid understanding;

+ have high expectations of all young people.

Demonstrating high expectations of refugees and asylum seekers demonstrates to them that their teachers care for them. This facilitates a sense of belonging and motivates them to work hard. All young people expect their teachers to have high expectations of them. It is essential that they are not identified as having special educational needs simply because they do not speak English. If teachers are concerned that a young person may have cognition and learning difficulties the assessment should be carried out in the child's home language to ascertain the child's level of development in comparison with their peers. Where difficulties in learning arise due to a language barrier, the young person does not have special educational needs. Their development has stunted because they cannot demonstrate their current level of achievement in English, not because they have a problem with learning. In these cases, young people should be provided with a new to English programme which will support their language development.

Opportunities should be provided for the young person to participate in a range of extracurricular activities. Again, this will aid social connectivity and language development. It will also facilitate a sense of belonging.

In 2017, over 2,500 separated children were referred to the Refugee Council's Children's Section. These children claim asylum in the UK, arriving alone, with no family to support them.

(Refugee Council: www.refugeecouncil.org.uk)

Research (Peterson et al, 2017) has found that young people who are asylum seekers or refugees demonstrate a strong commitment to education and schooling and have high aspirations for their futures, despite the existence of significant barriers to their educational pathways. Provision of educational guidance and counselling relating to pathways into higher education is not always available to asylum-seeking and refugee children, yet it provides a key mechanism for supporting educational transitions into higher education.

SUMMARY

This chapter has outlined the range of strategies aimed at helping those in care and care leavers, those who have experienced domestic abuse, those involved in gang-affiliated culture and finally asylum-seeking and refugee children. Services to which they can be signposted, and support that can be offered, have been outlined. The need for good therapeutic interventions has been a theme throughout and the need for joint collaborative action with other services is key.

CHECKLIST

This chapter has addressed:

✓ the need to involve other services to help provide effective mental health support;

✓ the importance of appropriate therapeutic services, such as CBT;

✓ the role you can play in helping young people experiencing mental health issues as a result of their wider upbringing and context.

FURTHER READING

Department for Education and Department of Health (2017) *Transforming Children and Young People's Mental Health Provision: A Green Paper.* London: DfE.

NSPCC (2018) *Children in Care,* NSPCC.

Redthread King's Youth Violence Project www.redthread.org.uk/projects/kings.

+ CHAPTER 6

SUPPORTING YOUNG PEOPLE WHO IDENTIFY AS LGBT+

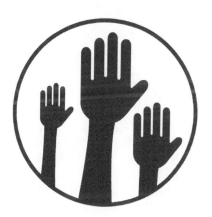

PROFESSIONAL LINKS

This chapter addresses the following Acts:

Human Rights Act 1998;

Equality Act 2010.

CHAPTER OBJECTIVES

By the end of this chapter you will understand:

+ the interplay between 'coming out' and mental health issues;

+ how to support inclusion for LGBT+ young people including developing an inclusive curriculum, using specialist services and protecting children at risk of harmful behaviour online;

+ where you can go for further advice.

INTRODUCTION

The Humans Right Act 1998 means that young people who identify as lesbian, gay, bisexual or transgender plus (LGBT+) are allowed to live their lives in the gender they feel is true for them, and that they should be protected from any degrading treatment, have a right to privacy about their gender or sexual identity, should be allowed to express themselves as they wish and should not be unfairly discriminated against.

The Equality Act 2010 means that students identifying as LGBT+ are legally protected against discrimination and Part Six of the Act makes specific reference to education and young people. It emphasises that to be protected by the Act, a young person is not required to be under-going any medical procedures but must simply be taking steps to live in the gender which they identify as, or are planning to do so. The Act also covers wider discrimination of the parents or siblings of the LGBT+-identifying person, which may arise as a result of their association with the individual.

This chapter outlines some of the ways in which the act of 'coming out' is often inextricably linked with mental health issues in a young person. It outlines some of the health challenges they face, including stress, major depressive disorder and suicidal feelings which many try to act upon.

This chapter also highlights areas where many schools, youth clubs and other child-related settings often fail in their legal duties to accommo-date LGBT+-identifying children which can lead to further mental health issues, and offers advice on how this can be prevented.

This chapter outlines how you can support the inclusion of LGBT+ young people and where you can find professional service teams who can provide further support where needed.

THE INTERPLAY BETWEEN 'COMING OUT' AND A YOUNG PERSON'S MENTAL HEALTH

Gender dysphoria is when a person experiences extreme distress due to a mismatch between their biological sex and gender identity. The clinical term has recently ceased to be classified as a mental disorder in itself (World Health Organization, 2018). This is because medical experts realised that gender dysphoria is not a mental health condition and calling it one can result in an increase in the risk of stigma to individuals who experience gender dysphoria. This change follows the way in which homosexuality ceased to be called a mental disorder relatively recently in 1992. Despite this, many gender diverse and transgender-identifying children and young people still suffer from a number of mental health issues that arise from the gender incongruence feelings they experience on a daily basis for a prolonged period of time. Many of these mental health issues are similar to those experienced by LGBT+-identifying children.

For most young people, the act of coming out can be a particularly challenging time in terms of managing their mental health and wellbeing. Initially, many have fears of family and friends rejecting them or other concerns about harassment at school or in other settings. However, one of the biggest and most traumatic issues for many children identifying as LGBT+ is that they are still coming to terms with their own gender/sexual identity. This can be, for some, harder than coming out to others as they process what this might mean for their future. Many experience self-hatred, suicidal feelings and a desire to self-harm (Bradlow et al, 2017). This can also lead to low attainment at school and a desire, which they regularly act upon, to skip school to avoid the bullying that they face.

Many young people know they are lesbian, gay or bisexual by the age of 11 or 12 years but often do not come out until they are 15 or 16 years old. This period has been called the **isolation years** and is the most vital time for directing support and information to those individuals.

- 52 per cent of bullied LGBT+ students feel that bullying has had a negative effect on their plans for future education, and 68 per cent of bullied trans children and young people also feel this way.

- 80 per cent of trans young people have self-harmed, as have 60 per cent of LGBT+ students.

- 92 per cent of trans young people have considered suicide and more than 40 per cent of trans young people have attempted to take their own life, as have 20 per cent of LGB-identifying young people.

- 45 per cent, including 64 per cent of trans pupils, are bullied for being LGBT+ in Britain's schools.

- 50 per cent of LGBT+ children and young people hear homophobic slurs 'frequently' or 'often' in schools.

- Just 20 per cent of trans young people have been taught about safe sex in relation to same-sex relationships.

(Bradlow et al, 2017)

CRITICAL QUESTIONS

+ What practical steps could you take to help improve some of the facts from the statistics box above in your work place this week?

+ What actions can schools take to provide a more supportive and inclusive environment for students who identify as LGBT+?

HOW TO SUPPORT INCLUSION FOR YOUNG PEOPLE IDENTIFYING AS LGBT+

DEVELOPING AN INCLUSIVE CURRICULUM

For many children and young people, how they see themselves, each other and their position in the world is formed by the knowledge they acquire and are taught in school. As mentioned in the introduction to this chapter, all public sector establishments are required by law to ensure that there is no discrimination to any child or young person identifying as LGBT+ on the grounds of their sexual orientation or gender identity. They also need to ensure that equality of opportunity is promoted and to take proper steps to ensure the promotion of different groups of individuals. If students identifying as LGBT+ are made to feel invisible and underrepresented in school, in terms of both their personal needs and the invisibility of the sexuality or gender identity group to which they identify with, this can heighten feelings of isolation and loneliness.

One way in which schools and youth centres can make the visibility of LGBT+ individuals clear is through creating an inclusive curriculum. Stonewall (Bradlow et al, 2017) recommends this can be done through ensuring that people who are LGBT+ are included in what is being taught, highlighting relevant things about them when they arise naturally, supporting staff through training to develop an inclusive vocabulary inclusive vocabulary, sharing ideas of how to better include LGBT+ content within the school's curriculum, sharing resources to help save time and providing opportunities for LGBT+ pupils to give their own suggestions about what to include. At the end of this chapter, links have been provided to offer subject-specific guidance for a wide range of subjects. Some recommended examples include the following.

+ For English, include books by authors and characters who are LGBT+, setting up speeches, discussions, and introducing writing activities on LGBT+ topics.

+ For maths, when teaching code breaking, explore the life of Alan Turing, who cracked the Enigma code during the Second World War and saved the lives of many people.

+ For science, highlight LGBT+ scientists and figures such as Francis Bacon or Louise Pearce and their contributions to the scientific, technical, engineering and medical fields.

+ For religious education, profile people of faith who are LGBT+, including English broadcaster and campaigner Vicky Beeching or Australia's only openly gay imam, Nur Warsame.

+ In the field of physical education, anti-LGBT+ abuse is often still common. An inclusive curriculum for physical education could include discussing equality, raising the profile of anti-homophobia in sports and highlighting sports people who identify as LGBT+. Additionally, it is important to emphasise to students that individuals who identify as LGBT+ can participate fully in all sports.

All students should be taught about the dangers and risks of 'do-it-yourself transitioning', otherwise known as when a young person may take sex hormones, which can cause many physiological and psychological health concerns if administered in unmonitored doses. Attempts to self-medicate are popular in trans-identifying young people who grow frustrated with long waiting lists to see gender specialists at gender identity clinics.

CRITICAL QUESTIONS

+ What are the challenges associated with updating a school's curriculum so that it is more LGBT+ inclusive for the children and young people who attend?

+ How might these challenges be overcome?

HIGH-QUALITY SEX AND RELATIONSHIPS EDUCATION

The UK government is committed to making age-appropriate relationships and sex education compulsory in all of England's schools in 2019, with amendments to the Children and Social Work Act 2017. Sex education will be renamed 'relationships education' in primary school settings and 'relationships and sex education' in secondary schools. This is the first time in which the sex education guidance has been edited since 2000 and clearly there have been significant changes in the last 18 years that must be addressed when delivering sex education to children and young people in the twenty-first century.

It is important that schools and centres working with children and young people offer inclusive relationship and sex advice. This is to ensure all children's and young people's identities and families are represented, and the learning needs of the children involved are met. Where staff working with children can 'miss the mark', it is often by assuming that all children are heterosexual, thus leaving those who identify as LGBT+ isolated and self-questioning as to whether their feelings are 'real' and 'normal', owing to the complete lack of information provided about their gender identity or sexual orientation.

Other assumptions, such as the assumption that all gay men will engage in anal sex or assumptions that all babies are conceived and born into the world in the same way, are often provided in class, but these ideas are now heavily outdated. This kind of teaching ignores different types of sex and reproduction, specifically other methods in which children are conceived and carried, for example, through in vitro fertilisation or surrogacy. It is important to address historical myths, such as HIV being a 'gay man's virus', as more heterosexual people now live with HIV than gay or bisexual men in the UK. Inclusive language should be used such as 'learners, students, Year 8', rather than single-sex terminology. The terms penis and vagina should be used instead of boys' parts or girls' parts to thoroughly include students of all gender identities or those transitioning. It is also important to remember that some screening procedures, such as cervical screening, may be important for trans men. More information about resources that can be signposted to those with responsibilities for the teaching of sex education in schools is included at the end of this chapter.

An inclusive sex education curriculum can help to alleviate some mental health problems such as stress around lack of invisibility or mental health issues that can be worsened through damage caused by a lack of awareness around staying safe and healthy in sex and relationships.

CRITICAL QUESTIONS

+ What are the dangers of the needs of children and young people who identify as LGBT+ not being addressed through high-quality inclusive sex education?

+ What reasonable steps could you take to prevent these dangers from happening?

HIGH-QUALITY COUNSELLING AND TALK THERAPIES

Many transgender young people will avoid situations that might expose them to harassment or discrimination. These situations may include schools or youth clubs, where young people should be able to access appropriate support. Young trans people and children may also dress in the gender role they feel is more 'passable', in order to be accepted, as opposed to the gender identity with which they identify internally. This can lead to significant distress and emotional chaos as they conceal their true identity and feelings. Other students may choose to attend a new school, college or youth group once they have transitioned, as a fresh start, but live in fear of others 'outing' them or their previous identity being disclosed unknowingly through word of mouth. There are physiological changes that can be particularly problematic and stressful for trans children, such as the pitch of their voice, which can disclose their identity, or painful physiological symptoms brought on from breast binding, which is where a trans boy may try to flatten the breasts using material, which can result in lung constriction and scarring. With so many psychological and physiological issues that LGBT+ people may need help with, one way in which schools and children's centres can help them is through setting up in-house counselling and therapeutic talk services. This provides them with the opportunity to discuss fears and concerns that they may be living with. There is plenty of advice available on the Department for Education's website on how to set up effective counselling in schools including advice on how to ensure that it runs in a professional and law-abiding way. More details are outlined at the end of the chapter.

PROTECTING AGAINST THE SIGNIFICANT RISKS POSED BY ONLINE BEHAVIOURS

The internet provides children and young people with fantastic opportunities to network with each other and help each other at particularly challenging times in their lives. However, as most of us are fully aware, the internet does have a dangerous side. With the widespread prevalence of pornography and an increase in young people creating sexualised images of themselves, young people find themselves at risk of sexual exploitation from predatory adults looking for vulnerable individuals to exploit. These risks are higher for LGBT+ young people, as they are often scared of being judged about their sexual orientation or identity and are less likely to discuss it with responsible adults that they know in person, and are therefore more likely to engage in interactions with strangers online.

For many young people, meeting strangers from the internet can be incredibly appealing, as it does not involve any of the threats that are often associated with direct social interactions. Kate Burls, Education Team Coordinator at the Child Exploitation and Online Protection (CEOP) Command, part of the National Crime Agency, has recently described sexting as the 'norm' for young people in their peer group. The House of Commons Education and Health Committees (2017) shared evidence that sexting, cyberbullying and inappropriate content have caused a direct increase in mental health problems in children, including stress and anxiety.

Under the Protection of Children Act 1978 and the Criminal Justice Act 1988, if a young person creates a sexually explicit image of themselves or someone else under the age of 18 years, they have created an indecent image of a child and receiving or sending this image equates to the possession or distribution of child pornography. Many young people identifying as LGBT+ who look to explore their sexual identity online, through sexting and sharing images of themselves, are at risk of illegal behaviour as a result. It is important to note that young people involved in sexting for the first time will not face criminal prosecution, but situations will be investigated to ensure that the young person is not at risk. When examples of sexting or images are shared, it can have devastating personal consequences, leading to humiliation, embarrassment and more abuse for young people who may already be experiencing mental ill health.

- Almost one in five under-18s identifying as LGBT+ has used adult dating apps such as Tinder, Grindr and Her.

- Two in five LGBT+ young people have met up with someone they met and talked to online. Of those, 30 per cent met someone older than them and 18 per cent did not tell anyone they were meeting up.

- More than two in five LGBT+ young people have sent or received sexual, naked or semi-naked photos to or from a person they were talking to online.

(Bradlow et al, 2017)

Those working to protect LGBT+ individuals from risky online behaviours need to share with them the impact that a casual approach to these kinds of risky activities can have on their lives. This is still a relatively under-researched area, but some research has shown that this kind of behaviour can lead to significantly increased suicidal feelings, depression, fear, poor self-confidence, lack of trust, being scared to go out and post-traumatic stress disorder. It can also lead to serious professional consequences, where young adults have had to leave jobs because of the fear of embarrassment or being frightened by a threat of what images will be published (Bond and Tyrell, 2018).

To protect the wellbeing of individuals identifying as LGBT+, who are vulnerable to these types of online sexual exploitation, important topics must be discussed with them to make them aware of these risks. Topics that should be covered to protect them include discussions around online grooming, oversharing, sexting and the use of smartphone apps and gaming sites where online criminals can target children and access their personal information such as their location. Children and young people in care who identify as LGBT+ may also be at further risk of unregulated contact with birth parents or relatives, when they may have entered care as a result of sexual abuse from these relatives, and of further cyberbullying.

There are online safety resources that can be discussed and shared available on the CEOP Command website, and the website address is given at the end of this chapter. These resources also show how you can report an incident to CEOP should you ever consider that it is necessary.

CRITICAL QUESTIONS

+ What signs might a child or young person who identifies as LGBT+ show that might reveal to you that they are engaging in risky online behaviours?

+ When dealing with these issues, which can be highly emotive and stressful for the responsible adult involved, how can you seek support for yourself?

CASE STUDY

'RISKING IT ANYWAY'

Ben was too ashamed to come out publicly at college, so he downloaded apps like Grindr and Scruff to find partners and friends. He was suddenly super excited that others were paying attention to his life. He forged new friendships but also began having online sexual relationships with others, some of whom he was not exactly sure how old they were. Soon he was spending ten hours a week on the sites and began to become addicted.

Over time, one user Ben talked to became more and more threatening. He said he was going to share all the explicit images Ben had sent him with all Ben's Facebook friends and family if he did not keep sending him more and more photos. Ben felt incredibly distressed but felt forced to continue doing it to prevent this from happening. His confidence was destroyed, he was ashamed with what he had done and felt isolated, lonely and suicidal.

Ben's youth worker Kamal noticed that Ben was suddenly behaving differently. He was staying away from the youth club and avoiding being alone with people, such as his family members and friends. He looked really tired and was showing signs of highly distraught behaviour. He seemed frightened to socialise all of a sudden. Kamal talked to him and eventually Ben opened up. Kamal reminded him of all the support available, including specialist abuse-related support. Kamal made the centre's Safeguarding Officer aware of his concerns about Ben's behaviour and actions. The police became involved after Ben and Kamal reported it together. The police investigated and managed to stop the culprit, and the perpetrator was prosecuted. Ben knew that he no longer had to suffer in silence and was beginning, over time, to feel mentally healthy. Had the youth worker not spotted the signs, this could have gone on for years, to the point where Ben may have acted on his suicidal feelings.

FURTHER ADVICE AND SPECIALIST SUPPORT

There are now significant numbers of advice and specialist support teams available to provide help to people who identify as LGBT+ and those who work with them. If you know a child or young person wanting more advice about transitioning, the NHS website has information about treatment for gender dysphoria and gender-confirmation surgery. This information can be found at www.nhs.uk/conditions/gender-dysphoria.

The charity Mind has a LGBT+-focused section featuring more information on those experiencing mental health problems as a result of their gender identity or sexuality, particularly those suffering from depression, anxiety and suicidal feelings. This expert help can be found at www.mind.org.uk.

For those considering coming out, the Proud Trust offers resources for everyone. These include some of the feelings that young people identifying as LGBT+ might have and how others can support them, so there is something in there for everyone. Visit www.theproudtrust.org for more information.

Stonewall has created documents full of advice for young people identifying as LGBT+. These include support needed to come out, stories, facts and tips. The Young Stonewall project was funded by the Department for Health's Sexual Identity and Gender Orientation Advisory Group and is a really accessible document. The document can be located at www. youngstonewall.org.uk. Stonewall also has a feature called 'What's on in my area?' This helps individuals to find LGBT+ and community groups that are local to them. This is a great resource for those wanting to form friendships with others who live nearby.

The Prince's Trust website has a database of helpful links to sites for those who also identify as LGBT+, disabled, the homeless or ex-offenders, to name a few. This can be located at www.princes-trust.org.

All Sorts Youth, a charity based in Brighton and Hove, listens to, supports and connects children and young people under 26 years. They also help to raise awareness, promote inclusion and facilitate safer and more supportive environments for LGBT+-identifying children and young people and do work in all areas of their lives. Their website can be found at www.allsortsyouth.org.

For parents and carers of children and young people identifying as LGBT+, the Stonewall website has a page of support and advice. This can be found at www.stonewall.org.uk.

For setting up an in-school counselling service, consult the Department for Education's *Counselling in Schools: A Blueprint for the Future* document, which is available at www.gov.uk/government/publications/counselling-in-schools.

For help with dealing with students at risk of child sexual exploitation, refer to the guidance and instructions found at www.ceop.police.uk and remember to always contact the school's or centre's Designated Safeguarding Lead in the first instance, who will be trained in dealing with such matters.

Before young people are signposted to external agencies, though, schools should signpost them to school-based services such as the school counselling service or the school wellbeing or pastoral team. Schools can also signpost young people to peer ambassadors who have received training to enable them to provide peer support.

SUMMARY

This chapter has outlined the impact coming out can have on a young person's mental health and wellbeing. The ways in which you can promote inclusive practice through the curriculum, talk therapies and protecting them from risks online have been described. The chapter has provided seven different recommended specialist support services.

CHECKLIST

This chapter has addressed the following:

✓ young people are at risk of serious mental ill health as a result of thinking about or actually coming out as LGBT+;

✓ schools must prioritise creating an inclusive curriculum to prevent further isolation and oppression of children and young people identifying as LGBT+;

✓ counselling and talk therapies can be very helpful in relieving some of the mental health symptoms;

✓ children identifying as LGBT+ are particularly at risk of participating in risky online behaviours that can result in mental ill health. Steps can be taken to prevent this from happening;

✓ there are specialist support services available to those needing help.

FURTHER READING

Barnes, E and Carlile, A (2018) *How to Transform Your School into an LGBT+ Friendly Place*. London: Jessica Kingsley.

Bradlow, J, Bartram F, Guasp, A and Jadva, V (2017) *School Report: The Experiences of Lesbian, Gay, Bi and Trans Young People in Britain's Schools in 2017*. London: Stonewall.

✚ CHAPTER 7

IDENTIFYING AND SUPPORTING YOUNG PEOPLE WHO EXPERIENCE BULLYING

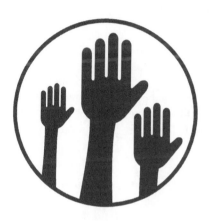

PROFESSIONAL LINKS

This chapter addresses the following:

The *Teachers' Standards* (2011) state that teachers have a professional duty to safeguard children and young people. This is one of the statutory responsibilities that schools must fulfil.

CHAPTER OBJECTIVES

By the end of this chapter you will understand:

+ what constitutes bullying;

+ how to identify bullying;

+ about evidence-based approaches for addressing bullying.

INTRODUCTION

All schools are legally required to have an anti-bullying policy. The school leadership team plays a critical role in establishing a whole-school culture that promotes the values of care, respect, kindness and inclusion for all members of the school community. This includes promoting an anti-bullying policy between members of staff. However, policies alone are insufficient. The values that policies promote must be borne out in practice.

The digital revolution and the popularity of social media have resulted in new forms of bullying. Bullying takes place online, outside the walls of the school. However, it impacts on relationships between young people in school. This chapter addresses the different forms of bullying that take place in schools and provides coverage of evidence-based strategies which can be adopted by schools as part of a whole-school approach to combatting bullying.

CRITICAL QUESTIONS

+ Do schools have a responsibility to address bullying between young people which takes place outside of school? Justify your response.

+ Do schools have a responsibility to support bullies as well as victims of bullies? Explain your response.

WHAT IS BULLYING?

The following definition of bullying is useful:

There is no legal definition of bullying. But it is usually defined as repeated behaviour which is intended to hurt someone either emotionally or physically and is often aimed at certain people because of their race, religion, gender or sexual orientation or any other aspect such as appearance or disability.

(BullyingUK, nd)

TYPES OF BULLYING

Bullying can take many forms, including:

+ *physical assault;*

+ *teasing;*

+ *isolating someone;*

+ *verbal bullying;*

+ *emotional bullying;*

+ *cyberbullying.*

Bullying includes:

+ *name calling;*

+ *making things up to get someone into trouble;*

+ *hitting, pinching, biting, pushing and shoving;*

+ *taking things away from someone;*

+ *damaging a person's belongings;*

+ *stealing someone's money;*

+ *isolating someone by taking their friends away from them (relational bullying);*

+ *posting insulting messages or spreading rumours;*

+ *threats and intimidation;*

+ *making silent or abusive phone calls;*

+ *sending offensive text messages;*

+ *frightening someone.*

(BullyingUK, nd)

PHYSICAL BULLYING

Physical bullying can take a range of forms. These include: hitting; pushing; tripping someone; slapping; spitting; stealing or destroying possessions, including books, clothing or lunch money. Perpetrators of physical bullying may bully for a variety of reasons, including to exert physical power over someone who they perceive to be weaker to gain control over the victim. They may have observed physical violence in the home. Perpetrators may have difficulty controlling their emotions.

VERBAL BULLYING

Verbal bullying is where someone directs verbal language towards another person with the intention of causing distress or embarrassment. While the effects of physical bullying might be immediately obvious, the effects of verbal bullying may not be immediately obvious. Girls tend to use verbal bullying rather than physical bullying. Perpetrators target victims for a range of reasons, including body image, clothing, social background, possessions, study habits, homophobia, disability and racism. The impact of this type of bullying can be significant. It can erode confidence and self-esteem and it can have a detrimental effect on attendance and academic attainment.

CRITICAL QUESTIONS

+ Why do you think that verbal bullying is more popular with girls than boys?
+ What do you think are the effects of verbal bullying?

SOCIAL AND EMOTIONAL BULLYING

Social and emotional bullying is sometimes referred to as relational bullying. Relational bullying refers to the harm that is caused within relationships, including friendships. It can be covert rather than overt and it can be manipulative. Examples of relational bullying include: social exclusion by separating someone from their friends; ignoring someone;

spreading rumours or gossip about someone and threatening someone if they do not comply with the wishes of the perpetrator.

Relational bullying can be difficult to address because perpetrators may feel that they are not breaking rules by ignoring someone. However, the impact on the victim can be significant. Again, it tends to be more common in girls than boys.

SEXUAL BULLYING

Sexual bullying is any bullying that has a sexual element. It can involve young people of any gender and it can also take place between young people and adults. Examples of sexual bullying include:

+ *sexual comments, taunts and threats;*

+ *inappropriate physical contact that makes the recipient feel uncomfortable or scared (this can include touching, 'up skirting', hugging and kissing);*

+ *distributing sexual material (including pornography);*

+ *'wolf-whistling';*

+ *sending photos or videos of a sexual nature;*

+ *making phone calls and sending texts or messages of a sexual nature;*

+ *'games' with a sexual element that may make a child or young person feel uncomfortable or scared (examples include taking clothes off, kissing or touching games);*

+ *pressure to spend time alone or apart from others with another person;*

+ *pressure to be in a relationship with another person, or to engage in a sexual act with another person, both inside and outside of school;*

+ *sexism in all its forms; pressure to conform to gender stereotypes.*

(Anti-bullying Alliance: www.anti-bullyingalliance.org.uk)

- 37 per cent of female students at mixed-sex schools have personally experienced some form of sexual harassment at school.

- 37 per cent of girls report experiencing sexual harassment, compared with 6 per cent of boys.

- 24 per cent of female students at mixed-sex schools have been subjected to unwanted physical touching of a sexual nature while at school.

- 32 per cent of teachers in mixed-sex secondary schools witness sexual harassment in their school on at least a weekly basis.

- 36 per cent of teachers say they witness it on a termly basis.

(www.teachers.org.uk)

SEXISM

Sexism is prejudice, stereotyping, or discrimination based on someone's sex. It can be a form of bullying when it is targeted at someone and is designed to cause distress or embarrassment.

- 66 per cent of female students and 37 per cent of male students in mixed-sex sixth forms have experienced or witnessed the use of sexist language in school.

- 64 per cent of teachers in mixed-sex secondary schools hear sexist language in school on at least a weekly basis.

- 29 per cent of teachers report that sexist language is a daily occurrence.

(www.teachers.org.uk)

HOMOPHOBIA, BIPHOBIA AND TRANSPHOBIA

Homophobia, biphobia or transphobia are types of bullying that take place because of a person's sexual orientation or gender identity. This

110

bullying contravenes the 2010 Equality Act, which identifies 'sexual orientation' and 'gender reassignment' as protected characteristics. The bullying can take a variety of forms including physical or verbal bullying, relational bullying, sexual bullying or cyberbullying. The use of homophobic, biphobic or transphobic language, even if dismissed as banter, also constitutes bullying. Young people who identify as transgender are particularly vulnerable to transphobic bullying.

Some young people who identify as LGBT+ do not experience a sense of belonging at home because they do not feel able to be open about their sexuality. If they come to school and experience homophobic, biphobic or transphobic bullying this can have a detrimental effect on their sense of belonging and this can result in poor mental health.

Stonewall's latest *School Report* (Bradlow et al, 2017), a study of over 3700 LGBT+ young people aged 11–19 years across the UK provides evidence on bullying of young people who identify as LGBT+. The key findings from Stonewall are alarming.

- 45 per cent of LGBT+ students are bullied for being LGBT+ at school.

- 64 per cent of trans pupils are bullied.

- 86 per cent of LGBT+ students regularly hear phrases such as 'that's so gay' or 'you're so gay' in school.

- 84 per cent of trans young people have self-harmed.

- 9 per cent of trans young people are subjected to death threats at school.

- 45 per cent of LGBT+ young people who are bullied for being LGBT+ never tell anyone about the bullying.

(Bradlow et al, 2017)

CRITICAL QUESTIONS

+ Why do you think people who are LGBT+ are vulnerable to being bullied?

+ What proactive strategies can schools adopt to promote inclusion for young people who identify as LGBT+?

+ What reactive strategies might schools adopt?

+ Young people who are bullied have a higher risk of mental health problems.

+ Persistent bullying can affect academic performance.

+ Persistent bullying can increase truancy.

+ Young people who are bullied are more likely to experience anxiety and depression.

(McDaid et al, 2017)

CASE STUDY

A secondary school developed a peer ambassador scheme to address bullying. The ambassadors were trained in different types of bullying and they were taught to recognise the signs of bullying. They ran a drop-in scheme to provide advice to young people who were experiencing bullying. They ran a helpline to provide victims of bullying with advice. At the end of the year, they organised a school conference on bullying. They developed a blog on bullying, which included a wide range of poems, personal accounts, artwork and photographs, which were all produced by students. They developed a display on bullying and contributed to the development of the personal and social education curriculum.

CRITICAL QUESTIONS

+ What are the ethical considerations in relation to this scheme?

+ How might you further develop the remit of the ambassadors?

RACISM

Racist bullying is abuse and harassment on the grounds of race, colour or beliefs. Racism is any incident which is perceived by a victim to be racist. Race, religion or belief are protected characteristics under the 2010 Equality Act. Schools therefore have a legal duty to prevent direct or indirect discrimination based on race, religion and belief.

DISABLIST BULLYING

Repetitive, intentional and hurtful behaviour targeted at individuals because they have a disability is disablist bullying. It can include physical and non-verbal bullying and includes the use of disablist language. Disablist bullying is discriminatory, oppressive or abusive behaviour targeted at people with disabilities. Perpetrators tend to believe that they are superior to people with disabilities and prejudice is often the root cause.

Reports suggest that bullying may have been experienced by:

- 80 per cent of young people with learning difficulties;
- 82 per cent of young people who have a stammer;
- 39 per cent of children with speech and language difficulties;
- almost 70 per cent of teachers have heard children using the words 'spaz', 'spastic', 'retard' or 'mong' at school;
- over 50 per cent of these teachers heard children using these words in 'casual' conversation; however, the same number heard them using the words as an insult to their peers;
- 55 per cent of teachers have heard children using the words to a child who is disabled or has special educational needs – with just under 50 per cent of them using the words to insult them;
- additionally, over 90 per cent of parents of children with Asperger's syndrome reported that their child had been bullied in the previous 12 months alone.

(Anti-bullying Alliance: www.anti-bullyingalliance.org.uk)

CYBERBULLYING

Cyberbullying is bullying which takes place over the internet, including bullying which takes place on social media. It takes a variety of forms. These include:

+ posting hurtful comments;
+ posting videos targeted directly at a person to cause distress;

+ posting photographs designed to cause distress;

+ inciting others to make hurtful comments aimed at a person;

+ sending hurtful text messages using a mobile phone;

+ sending hurtful private messages to a person.

This is not an exhaustive list and forms of cyberbullying are likely to expand as new applications and software are developed. Cyberbullying is fundamentally different to face-to-face bullying in several ways. First, victims cannot escape from the bullying when they are at home because it takes place on mobile phones, tablets and computers. Second, the abuse is witnessed by a larger audience; messages are in the public domain and can be repeatedly forwarded. This can result in victims experiencing the abuse on multiple occasions, which results in further psychological distress. Third, the evidence of the abuse is usually permanently stored online, which means that the abuse is not erased. These messages serve as a permanent reminder of the abuse and this can result in abuse being continually experienced by the victim.

Most social network sites have clear anti-bullying policies. However, social media companies have been slow to intervene in cases of abuse and in many instances, abuse has been left unchallenged. The growth in technology has enabled young people to stay in constant contact with each other. While this can be positive, it can also result in young people becoming victims of abuse.

One key question is 'what constitutes abuse?' Have you ever received a text message or an email and interpreted it differently to the person who sent it? Have you sometimes thought that someone was being nasty in a message and been upset by it, only to discover that that was not how the sender intended to make you feel? We interpret the information we receive in text via technology without other cues which are useful in communication. These include body language and tone of voice. Sometimes we may feel that another person is trying to hurt us via a message, but they may not have intended that. The critical point here is that users of technology must be taught to use it responsibly. We should carefully consider how a message might be perceived by the recipient before we send it, and whether there is any potential for causing distress. This is part of being a responsible user of technology. It is critical to the development of digital citizenship that every digital citizen understands how to use technology in a responsible way so as not to cause distress in others. Schools should include this as part of the digital curriculum. The important point to emphasise here is that regardless of whether an individual was not intending to cause harm or distress, if the recipient of a messages feels that they were being bullied and experiences distress, this constitutes cyberbullying.

Have you ever sent an email to someone which was then forwarded on to others? Or have you sent an email to someone who subsequently replied to you but copied others into the reply? Have you accidently received a confidential email that was intended for someone else? Have you ever been 'told off' by someone in an email but had others copied into the message? If you have answered 'yes' to these questions, how did this make you feel? If you experienced distress, anxiety or embarrassment, this might constitute cyberbullying. Responsible email use is essential. So that messages cannot be misinterpreted, it is important that forms of electronic communication are clear, concise and do not have the potential to cause harm.

HARASSMENT

Harassment is the act of sending offensive, rude, and insulting messages and being abusive. It includes nasty or humiliating comments on posts, photographs and in chat rooms, and making offensive comments on gaming sites. Posting false and malicious things about people on the internet can be classed as harassment.

DENIGRATION

Denigration is when someone may send information about another person that is fake, damaging and untrue. It includes sharing photographs of someone to ridicule and spreading fake rumours and gossip. This can be on any site online or on apps. It includes purposely altering photographs of others to ridicule and cause distress.

FLAMING

Flaming is when someone purposely uses extreme and offensive language and deliberately gets into online arguments and fights. They do this to deliberately cause distress in others.

115

IMPERSONATION

Impersonation is when someone hacks into someone's email or social networking account and uses the person's online identity to send or post vicious or embarrassing material to or about others. It also includes making up fake profiles of others.

OUTING AND TRICKERY

Outing and trickery is when someone shares personal information about someone else or tricks someone into revealing secrets and subsequently forwards them to others. They may also do this with private images and videos too.

CYBERSTALKING

Cyberstalking is the act of repeatedly sending messages that include threats of harm, harassment, intimidating messages, or engaging in other online activities that make a person afraid for their safety. The actions may be illegal depending on what they are doing. Cyberstalking can take place on the internet or via mobile phones. Examples include:

+ silent calls;
+ insulting and threatening texts;
+ abusive verbal messages;
+ cases of stolen identities.

EXCLUSION

Exclusion is when others intentionally leave someone out of a group, such as group messages, online apps, gaming sites and other online engagement. This is also a form of social bullying and is very common.

SPREADING RUMOURS AND GOSSIP

Online abuse, rumours and gossip can go viral very quickly and can be shared by many people within several minutes. It is not uncommon for former close friends or partners to share personal secrets about victims.

THREATENING BEHAVIOUR

Threatening behaviour directed at a victim to cause alarm and distress is a criminal offence. Taking screenshots of the evidence and reporting it is one way of challenging this.

HAPPY SLAPPING

Happy slapping is an incident where a person is assaulted while other people take photographs or videos on their mobile phones. The pictures or videos are then circulated by mobile phone or uploaded on the internet.

GROOMING

Grooming is when someone builds an emotional connection with a child to gain their trust for the purposes of abuse and exploitation. It is conducted by strangers (or new 'friends') and may include:

+ pressurising someone to do something they do not wish to do;

+ making someone take their clothes off;

+ pressurising someone to engage in sexual conversations;

+ pressurising someone to take naked photographs of themselves;

+ making someone engage in sexual activity via the internet.

Groomers may spend a long time establishing a 'relationship' with the victim by using the following strategies:

+ *pretending to be someone they are not, for example saying they are the same age online;*

+ *offering advice or understanding;*

+ *buying gifts;*

+ *giving the child attention;*

+ *using their professional position or reputation;*

+ *giving compliments;*

+ *taking them on trips, outings or holidays.*

(NSPCC: www.nspcc.org.uk)

It is against the law for anyone under the age of 18 years to take, send or redistribute pictures of anyone under the age of 18 years. Groomers can be male or female and they can be of any age.

The Child Exploitation and Online Protection Command investigates cases of sexual abuse and grooming on the internet.

INAPPROPRIATE IMAGES

It is very easy to save any pictures of anyone on any site and upload them to the internet. Uploading pictures of someone to cause distress is a form of cyberbullying. This also includes digitally altering pictures to embarrass someone.

BYSTANDER EFFECT

Witnessing cyberbullying and doing nothing about it is not acceptable. Some people are worried about getting involved but victims of bullying need brave witnesses to make a stand. Perpetrators of bullying thrive when they have an audience. Making a stand against what they are doing is a key way to reduce their power. Most sites operate a reporting facility so that online abuse can be reported and addressed. Bystanders are not innocent. They have a responsibility to report abuse that they witness.

(www.bullying.co.uk)

CRITICAL QUESTIONS

+ Have you experienced cyberbullying?

+ If so, what form(s) did it take?

+ How did it affect you?

SIGNS OF CYBERBULLYING

Signs of cyberbullying include:

+ *low self-esteem;*

+ *withdrawal from family and spending a lot of time alone;*

+ *reluctance to let parents or other family members anywhere near their technological devices;*

+ *finding excuses to stay away from school or work, including school refusal;*

+ *friends disappearing or being excluded from social events;*

+ *losing weight or changing appearance to try and fit in;*

+ *fresh marks on the skin that could indicate self-harm and dressing differently, such as wearing long-sleeved clothes in the summer to hide any marks;*

+ *a sudden change in behaviour; that is, anger, depression, crying, withdrawal.*

(BullyingUK: www.bullying.co.uk)

Signs could also include:

+ *anxiousness;*

+ *clingy behaviour;*

+ *depression;*

+ *aggressive behaviour;*

+ *difficulties sleeping;*

+ *wetting the bed;*

+ *soiled clothes;*

+ *risk-taking behaviour;*

+ *obsessive behaviour, including constantly checking their phone;*

+ *nightmares;*

+ *substance abuse;*

+ *self-harm;*

+ *thoughts about suicide.*

(NSPCC: www.nspcc.org.uk)

THE EFFECTS OF CYBERBULLYING

According to the Royal Society for Public Health:

*Victims of bullying are more likely to experience low academic perform-
ance, depression, anxiety, self-harm, feelings of loneliness and changes
in sleeping and eating patterns – all of which could alter the course of a
young person's life as they undertake important exams at school or university and develop personally and socially.*

(Royal Society for Public Health, 2017, p 11)

Childhood bullying can have long-lasting and permanent effects. It can
lead to diminished confidence and poor self-esteem and these can
have a detrimental effect on academic performance.

● Seven in ten young people have experienced cyberbullying.

● 37 per cent of young people experience cyberbullying on a
frequent basis.

● Young people are twice as likely to be bullied on Facebook than
on any other social network.

● 91 per cent of young people who reported cyberbullying said
that no action was taken.

(Royal Society for Public Health, 2017)

CRITICAL QUESTIONS

+ Why do you think the statistics for cyberbullying are so high?

+ What type of bullying is worse – cyberbullying or traditional face-to face bullying?

The *Life in 'Likes'* research reported the following.

+ Cyberbullying was the most talked about issue in relation to the theme of 'what counts as safety?'

+ Many young people report that, when faced with cyberbullies, they knew to ignore the comments and remind themselves that the bully must be 'jealous' or 'insecure'.

+ Many young people felt confused whether a mean comment someone writes to them was real or a joke.

+ Many young people were uncomfortable when they saw content that was racist or violent.

(Children's Commissioner, 2018)

BULLYING OR BANTER?

Some young people dismiss unacceptable comments towards others as 'banter'. Young people need to be supported to understand the impact that words and phrases can have on other people. Schools need to help young people to understand that regardless of whether they intended to hurt someone else, if someone perceives that they are being bullied then the school has a responsibility to treat it as a bullying case. Some young people pass off homophobic remarks as banter through using phrases such as 'that bag is gay'. The problem here is that the word 'gay' is being used as a synonym for 'rubbish' and therefore the use of the word gay in this context can cause distress, even though that may not have been the intention of the person who used the word.

WHAT STRATEGIES CAN SCHOOLS USE TO ADDRESS BULLYING?

SCHOOL CULTURE AND ETHOS

The school leadership team plays a critical role in creating a positive school culture which engenders a sense of belonging in all members of the school community. The approach should include:

+ promoting, valuing and celebrating diversity;

+ challenging banter;

+ creating a climate of respect for all;

+ engendering a culture in which everyone knows that it is not only wrong to 'say it' but it is wrong to even 'think it';

+ ensuring that everyone is safe;

+ ensuring a mutual commitment to caring for others and keeping others safe;

+ establishing a zero-tolerance line on bullying, discrimination and harassment;

+ promoting a culture that empowers everyone to challenge and report bullying.

PEER MENTORING

Peer mentors are paired with a designated mentee. They provide support through offering a 'drop-in' service to vulnerable peers.

PEER LISTENING AND COUNSELLING

Young people are more likely to tell a peer about problems than an adult. Peer listeners are older students who provide a listening ear for students who need advice and emotional support.

PEER MEDIATION

Some schools operate a peer mediation service. Peer mediators are trained in conflict resolution strategies and they help perpetrators and victims to resolve issues.

BUDDY SCHEMES

Peer buddies provide targeted social and emotional support to vulnerable young people. Older peers are usually matched with younger students. Buddies may also have previous experience of bullying and mental health problems and these problems may have been resolved. Their experiences provide them with a solid grounding to support their peers who may be experiencing similar problems.

CIRCLE OF FRIENDS

Volunteer pupils are trained to befriend and support other pupils who are identified as isolated or rejected by their peers. They meet as a group with a teacher to discuss ways of supporting the vulnerable peer. They allocate roles and responsibilities so that these are distributed across the volunteers.

CYBER MENTORS

Cyber mentors are trained to provide online support and advice to peers. Communication may be through an online chat room or via text message.

BYSTANDER TRAINING

All young people could potentially be witnesses of bullying. Young people should be educated through personal and social education about different types of bullying so that they can recognise it when it occurs. They should be taught about the impact of bullying on others and their responsibilities in relation to bullying when they witness it.

TELLING SCHOOLS

The school culture should promote a 'telling' culture, which emphasises the importance of reporting inappropriate behaviour when it is witnessed. All young people have a responsibility to challenge and report bullying when they see it. They belong to a school community in which everyone is responsible for the safety of other people.

PLAYGROUND CHARTERS

Some schools have developed playground charters, which set out the 'rules' for playground behaviour. These are generally more effective if young people have ownership of them by contributing to their development.

CLOSED-CIRCUIT TELEVISION

Some schools have invested in closed-circuit television (CCTV) as a mechanism to keep young people safe. This is based on the general assumption that young people will modify their behaviour if they know that they are being observed.

CRITICAL QUESTIONS

+ What are the ethical issues associated with the use of CCTV in schools?
+ What are the advantages of CCTV?
+ What are the disadvantages of CCTV?

RESTORATIVE APPROACHES

Restorative approaches focus on the resolution of conflict between the perpetrator and the victim of bullying. In this approach, the perpetrator and the victim meet face to face. The perpetrator is required to listen to the victim. The victim explains how the bullying affected them and other people, and what needs to happen to resolve the situation. In restorative approaches, the following aspects are being restored:

+ relationship, and even friendship;

+ empathy and respect;

+ understanding the impact of one's own behaviour on others;

+ sense of security;

+ self-confidence;

+ self-respect;

+ dignity.

The approach relies on honesty and unconditional positive regard for both the victim and the perpetrator. It is not a further opportunity to chastise the perpetrator. The approach is underpinned by the branch of psychology known as humanism. Humanism is underpinned by the work of Carl Rogers, who emphasised the importance of developing the sense of 'self'. The approach aims to develop a positive sense of self in both the perpetrator and the victim.

CRITICAL QUESTIONS

+ Are perpetrators of bullying also victims?

+ What are the benefits of a restorative approach?

+ What are the disadvantages of a restorative approach?

CURRICULUM

Young people need a curriculum which addresses bullying. This is usually taught through personal and social education. However, where possible, it should also be integrated through the curriculum. Examples are:

+ Cyberbullying can be addressed in computing.

+ The theme of bullying can be addressed in history when discussing the behaviours of famous people throughout history.

+ In English, the theme of bullying can be addressed through discussion of characters' behaviours in texts. Students can also write poems or stories about bullying.

REACTIVE APPROACHES

Schools tend to adopt reactive approaches for addressing bullying. These approaches ensure that bullying incidents are reported, addressed through applying sanctions and followed through by notifying parents. Schools must keep accurate records of bullying and these are reviewed by Ofsted during school inspections. Having a clear policy on sanctions is part of a reactive approach. While these reactive approaches are necessary, it is also important that schools address bullying using proactive approaches such as the ones discussed above.

SIGNPOSTING YOUNG PEOPLE

Research the following organisations or websites and consider whether you would recommend them to young people:

+ Kidscape: www.kidscape.org.uk.

+ Anti-bullying Alliance: www.anti-bullyingalliance.org.uk.

+ Childline: https://bounce-back-from-bullying.childline.org.uk.

+ BIRMINGHAM Police and Schools Panels, Bullying Resources and Signposting: http://policeandschools.org.uk/KNOWLEDGE%20 BASE/bullying.html.

+ BullyingUK: www.bullying.co.uk.

Before young people are signposted to external agencies, however, schools should signpost them to school-based services such as the school counselling service or the school wellbeing or pastoral team. Schools can also signpost young people to peer ambassadors who have received training to enable them to provide peer support.

SUMMARY

This chapter has introduced you to different types of bullying that you may see in secondary schools. We have explained what constitutes different types of bullying and we have presented some practical strategies that can be used as part of a whole-school approach to anti-bullying.

CHECKLIST

This chapter has addressed:

✓ that bullying takes a range of forms;

✓ that bullying can result in mental ill health;

✓ the importance of school culture in minimising bullying;

✓ evidence-based strategies to address bullying.

FURTHER READING

DeWolf, K A (2014) *Stop Bullying: Effective Ways to Overcome Bullying In School Permanently: Modern Day Approach To Prevent Bullying Once And For All*. Kindle edition; published through CreateSpace Independent Publishing Platform.

Thorsborne, M and Blood, P (2013) *Implementing Restorative Practices in Schools: A Practical Guide to Transforming School Communities*. London: Jessica Kingsley.

✚ CHAPTER 8

SUPPORTING MENTAL HEALTH NEEDS BY WORKING IN PARTNERSHIP

PROFESSIONAL LINKS

This chapter addresses the following:

The special educational needs and disabilities code of practice emphasises the importance of schools involving young people and parents in all decision-making processes and the importance of effective multi-agency collaboration.

CHAPTER OBJECTIVES

By the end of this chapter you will understand:

+ ways of working in partnership with young people, parents and external services to meet a young person's mental health needs;

+ current issues in relation to partnership working.

INTRODUCTION

Schools are well placed to support young people's mental health needs. They work with young people daily, and teachers are in a unique position to notice changes in mood and behaviour which may indicate there is a mental health need. Teachers are well placed to notice deteriorating attendance, progress and attainment, which may indicate that there is a problem. However, despite this, it is important to remember that teachers are not specialists in mental health. Working in partnership with young people, parents and other organisations enables teachers to more effectively meet the needs of young people. We are working in challenging economic times. Financial cuts to services have resulted in larger caseloads for counsellors, educational psychologists and mental health workers, and waiting times can be lengthy. This means that young people do not always receive the support they need at the point when they need it. This chapter explores approaches to partnership working and identifies some of the associated challenges.

EFFECTIVE PARTNERSHIP WORKING

Working in partnership with other stakeholders is complex, rewarding and challenging. Effective collaboration is dependent upon several factors. These include the following.

+ Child first: placing the young person central to the collaboration by focusing on outcomes for them helps to ensure that all decisions are made in the young person's best interests.

+ Knowledge: having knowledge of the roles and responsibilities of other professionals is essential to effective multi-agency collaboration.

+ Trust: trusting other professionals to fulfil their professional commitments within resource constraints will make it easier to establish mutual respect.

+ Communication: communicating clearly by avoiding discipline-specific language will help to establish a common language that everyone understands.

+ Respect: respecting other people's roles and adopting the guiding principle that all roles are of equal value will frame the way you treat other colleagues.

+ Professional boundaries: accepting that there are limits to one's professional role and that support from another professional or service team might be necessary when the limit has been reached.

WORKING IN PARTNERSHIP WITH YOUNG PEOPLE

Mental health is classed as a special educational need in the *Special Educational Needs and Disabilities Code of Practice* (Department for Education and Department of Health, 2015). One of the principles of this framework is that young people should be provided with opportunities to participate in decision-making processes. Involving young people in decisions that affect them is empowering and builds confidence and self-esteem. Young people have a unique knowledge of their needs and often can share insights into what strategies might help them.

THE UNITED NATIONS CONVENTION ON THE RIGHTS OF THE CHILD

Article 12 of the United Nations Convention on the Rights of the Child (UNCRC) states that every young person has the right to express their views, feelings and wishes in all matters affecting them, and to have their views considered and taken seriously. This right applies at all times. Article 13 states that every young person must be free to express their thoughts and opinions and to access all kinds of information, providing that it is within the law. The UNCRC is the most widely ratified human rights treaty in the world. The Convention came into force in the UK in 1992.

STUDENT VOICE

According to Public Health England (2015), 'Involving students in decisions that impact on them can benefit their emotional health and wellbeing by helping them to feel part of the school and wider community and to have some control over their lives' (p 14). Schools should ensure that young people have appropriate channels for expressing their views. They should be consulted about the curriculum, learning and teaching, behaviour and assessment policies, so that they can influence developments which may impact on their wellbeing. Schools should provide opportunities for young people to shape the development of the mental health curriculum and to lead on mental health through the introduction of peer mentoring or student ambassador schemes.

PEER MENTORING

Young people generally prefer to talk to other young people about their needs rather than talking to adults. One way of facilitating this is to develop peer mentoring. Peer mentoring can be implemented using a variety of approaches.

+ Young people can be paired. Mental health champions can be recruited to be peer mentors and they are subsequently matched to a peer to provide them with a 'listening ear'. This can work well, as it can provide a vulnerable young person with emotional support.

+ Mental health champions can be trained in mental health needs and they are subsequently deployed to run 'drop-in' sessions which vulnerable young people access.

CRITICAL QUESTIONS

+ What are the attributes of a good peer mentor?

+ What criteria would you use to select peer mentors?

+ What training would peer mentors need in ethical practice?

+ What are the benefits of peer mentoring to mentors and mentees?

+ What are the limitations of peer mentoring?

IDENTIFYING NEEDS AND MONITORING IMPACT

Identification of needs in schools is often unsystematic and relies on young people demonstrating symptoms. Once these symptoms have been identified, the need is then targeted through intervention programmes to address it. However, many young people who have mental health needs do not demonstrate visible symptoms of a need. This means that needs may not be identified and may go unaddressed.

The *Special Educational Needs and Disabilities Code of Practice* (Department for Education and Department of Health, 2015) states that young people must be provided with opportunities to participate in decision-making processes. Schools should involve young people in the initial assessment of their needs through seeking their perspectives. Young people should also be involved in reviewing their own progress regularly and their perspectives on the effectiveness of interventions should be sought. Additionally, young people should participate in setting goals or targets and identify ways through which they can achieve them.

The characteristics of effective peer mentoring schemes have been identified in several research studies.

+ Co-production of schemes by young people in the school support the effectiveness of peer mentoring (Houlston and Smith, 2009).

+ Distributing the leadership of schemes is important, so that the commitments do not all fall on a single person (Cowie and Wallace, 2000).

+ The senior leadership team must commit to the scheme (Parsons et al, 2008).

CASE STUDY

A secondary school recruited ten mental health champions. The school developed clear criteria for selection and they operated a recruitment process which included a letter of application and a face-to-face interview. Once selected, the peer mentors completed a training course in mental health. The peer mentors completed a range of tasks during the year. They produced guidance leaflets for their peers on different aspects of mental health, with advice on how to manage specific needs such as anxiety and depression. They ran confidential drop-in sessions at lunchtime for their peers. They contributed to the development of the mental health curriculum for all students in Year 8 and they led some of these sessions. Finally, they organised a student-led mental health conference. This was entirely led by students and included presentations, drama, artwork, poetry, film making and music.

CRITICAL QUESTIONS

+ What are the risks associated with young people producing guidance for their peers on mental health?

+ How might you develop the role of the student mental health champion if you are asked to lead on this?

PARTNERSHIPS WITH PARENTS

Another principle in the code of practice is that schools are required to increase parental participation in supporting their child's needs. Schools are required to include the perspectives of parents in decision-making processes. Parents can participate in the initial identification of their child's mental health needs, setting targets and in reviewing their child's progress.

THE MENTAL HEALTH NEEDS OF PARENTS

Some young people who have mental health needs also have parents who have mental health needs. These needs may have prevented them from forming secure attachments with their child. Additionally, in some cases, where parents display mental health needs their children may end up caring for their parent and the parent may lack capacity to adequately care for their child. In some cases, the needs of some parents are so serious that they are unable to provide their child with a safe, caring and loving environment and, in these cases, schools may have no choice but to refer the matter to social care. The decision to take children into care should always be a last resort. In some cases, young people who have parents with mental health needs end up becoming young carers for their parents and this can result in mental health needs developing in the young person. Schools have a duty of care to ensure that young people are protected from abuse and neglect. However, in many cases parents with mental health needs can provide their child with a loving, caring, stable and nurturing environment. It is important that schools adopt a non-judgemental stance towards parents with mental health needs. Teachers and senior leaders should demonstrate empathy and kindness towards all parents, but particularly towards those who are the most vulnerable.

Schools can support young people whose parents have mental health needs by providing access to pastoral support. The pastoral support worker is a point of contact for a young person; it is someone in whom the young person can confide when situations become difficult at home. Some young people may prefer to confide in a peer rather than talking to an adult. Peer mentoring can be effective in these situations. Where peer mentoring is used, it is essential that a positive, trusting relationship is established between the mentor and the mentee. The arrangement will need to be reviewed on a regular basis to check that it is working. Schools can support parents with mental health needs by signposting them to services in the community that can offer them support and by providing them with workshops on a variety of themes including:

+ stress management;

+ anger management;

+ ways of developing positive interactions with their children;

+ strategies for managing depression;

+ strategies for dealing with anxiety.

Approximately one in six adults in England reported experiencing a mental health problem in the last week.

Over two million children are estimated to be living with a parent who has a common mental health disorder.

(NSPCC: www.nspcc.org.uk)

IDENTIFYING NEEDS IN PARTNERSHIP WITH PARENTS

During the process of identifying mental health needs, it is important for schools to capture information about the young person's wellbeing outside school. This will help you to ascertain whether the mental health need is specific to the school context or whether it is evident outside school. You may have concerns about a young person. You may have noticed changes in their mood or behaviour. You may have recognised that the young person is demonstrating signs of anxiety or depression. You may have noticed that the young person is self-harming. They may suddenly have become withdrawn and tearful. Their attendance and academic profile may have started to decline. These are warning signs for further investigation.

After discussing your concerns with the young person, it might be necessary for you to meet with parents to discuss your concerns and to seek their perspectives. However, a decision to involve parents should only be taken after you have considered whether this will place the young person at risk of harm. You should explain to the young person why you need to involve their parents and what information you will share with them.

PARENTAL PARTICIPATION IN SETTING GOALS

It is important to help parents to understand that they have a role to play in establishing goals for their child and supporting their child to achieve these goals. They should be asked to contribute to goal setting, particularly by identifying goals for their child outside of school. It is important to help parents to recognise that goals do not always have to focus on academic aspirations. Goals can relate to social, physical or emotional wellbeing and parents may need support in understanding how these aspects relate to mental health. Once goals are identified you can work with parents to identify ways in which they can support their child to meet these.

PARENTAL PARTICIPATION IN REVIEWING PROGRESS

Systems should be in place to ensure that parents or carers are regularly updated on their child's progress and given opportunities to share

136

their perspectives. Effective provision goes beyond merely updating parents about their child's progress. Parents should be actively involved in contributing to progress reviews.

CRITICAL QUESTIONS

+ What are your views on the role of schools in supporting parents with mental health needs?

+ Approaches for working with parents may vary according to parental circumstances and the needs of the young person. Can you think of instances where the school may need to be more detached from parents to address a young person's mental health needs?

In a survey completed by over 1000 parents, the following key findings were identified:

+ 66 per cent of parents said a significant issue was waiting times;

+ 49 per cent of parents said no one believed them that there was a problem;

+ 36 per cent of parents said that they had paid private counsellors, psychologists or other therapists;

+ 41 per cent of parents felt excluded by the agencies involved in helping their young people;

+ parents wanted more practical advice on how to successfully navigate crises and avoid escalating the situation;

+ parents wanted schools to provide parent support workers as a point of contact;

+ parents requested more consistent crisis support, including out-of-hours support, telephone support lines and information on what to do in different situations.

(Association for Young People's Health, 2016)

CASE STUDY

A secondary school ran a series of workshops for parents to support them in managing their child's mental health needs. Topics included: managing stress, anxiety and depression at home; social media and mental health; self-harm; mindfulness and relaxation; and managing behaviour. Parents were given strategies that they could use at home with their child. All the attendees were mothers. All of them declared that they also used the strategies on themselves as well as with their child.

CRITICAL QUESTIONS

+ Are there any themes which should not be addressed in parental workshops and why?

+ How could the school have engaged fathers in this project?

+ Why do you think that fathers were reluctant to engage in this project?

PARTNERSHIPS WITH EXTERNAL AGENCIES INCLUDING THE VOLUNTARY SECTOR

Working in partnership with external agencies is essential when supporting a child with mental health problems. You need to understand the roles and responsibilities of different services and some of the challenges associated with multi-agency collaboration. The Mental Health Green Paper states that:

There is significant variation in access to children and young people's mental health services. Waits for treatment can vary considerably, in one area to another, with the shortest around four weeks and the longest in one area up to 100 weeks from referral to treatment.

(Department for Education and Department of Health, 2017: para 83, p 23)

Some young people can only access support when it is too late. The average waiting time in 2016–17 was 12 weeks (Department for Education and Department of Health, 2017). Other key issues are stated below.

+ Information about young people is not always shared efficiently between agencies.

+ It is often difficult to find a convenient time for different services to meet.

+ Different services do not always share a common language.

+ Specific services do not always feel valued by other services.

However, despite these issues, where multi-agency collaboration is working well, young people receive the support that they need, and they thrive. There is inequity in access to services across the country. This results in a postcode lottery with some young people getting the support they need while others are neglected.

THE ROLE OF CHILD AND ADOLESCENT MENTAL HEALTH SERVICES

Child and adolescent mental health services (CAMHS) provide specialist support for children with mental health needs. Local CAMHS are multi-professional teams which include a range of professionals. These include psychiatrists, psychologists, social workers, nurses, support workers, occupational therapists, psychological therapists (child psychotherapists, family psychotherapists, play therapists and creative art therapists), primary mental health link workers and specialist substance misuse workers. Schools can make referrals to CAMHS, but this provision is usually reserved for young people who have severe, complex and enduring difficulties. Schools will need to check referral criteria before contacting CAMHS and any decision to refer children for support must be taken with full agreement from the child's parents. Waiting times to access CAMHS can be lengthy and this can result in young people receiving help far too late. CAMHS do not provide support for young people solely with learning difficulties or for behavioural problems that are evident in school but not at home. They are specialist services for children and young people with severe, complex and enduring mental health needs.

REFERRALS TO CAMHS

CAMHS across England are operating within a period of significant budget cuts and waiting lists are lengthy. Before you take the decision to refer a young person to your local CAMHS, it is important to be familiar with the criteria for referral. Although each local service publishes its own criteria, there are some general guiding principles that you will need to consider before making a referral. These include:

+ the severity of the need;

+ the complexity of the need;

+ the duration of the need.

In relation to severity of need, you will need to consider how serious the problem is. Some problems are life-threatening or place the young person at risk of harm and these will need an immediate referral. Generally, CAMHS will only deal with cases that are severe. Examples include:

+ severe depression;

+ severe anxiety;

+ risk of suicide;

+ risk of self-harm or danger;

+ eating disorders;

+ obsessive compulsive disorders;

+ gender identity needs;

+ severe attachment needs.

This is not an exhaustive list. It merely illustrates a range of needs, which may be severe. Young people may present other needs that you consider to be severe. In relation to severity, you will need to consider the impact of the need on the child's mental health and overall life outcomes.

You will also need to take into account the complexity of the child's need(s). Complex needs arise from multiple risk factors. Specific groups are more at risk than others of developing mental health needs. These include:

+ children and young people who are socially disadvantaged;

+ looked-after children;

+ young people who identify as lesbian, gay, bisexual or transgender;

+ those not in education or training;

+ young people at risk of, or suffering, abuse, neglect, exploitation or youth violence, witnessing domestic abuse, being a young carer, or having a disability;

+ young carers;

+ young people who are in contact with the criminal justice system.

If young people fall into any one of these categories, they may present complex mental health needs. However, young people may fit into more than one of these categories and this can result in multiple needs which are complex to address and require specialist intervention.

You will need to consider the duration of the problem. Some CAMHS will only accept referral cases where the need has been evident for more than three months. However, judgements about whether a specific need is enduring should be balanced against the potential for harm to the child. It is possible that a mental health need may be so serious that it requires immediate referral to specialist services.

In all cases where teachers or other colleagues have concerns about a young person, the designated safeguarding lead in the school should be consulted as they are the person who will usually make the referral. The headteacher and other senior leaders may also need to be consulted. However, when making a referral it is important only to inform those people who need to know. The young person's rights to privacy and con- fidentiality should be respected but also balanced against the need to inform relevant people to mitigate risk of harm.

● There are approximately 460,000 referrals per year to children and young people's mental health services.

● 200,000 of these go on to receive treatment.

● In 2016/17 the average wait for treatment in a children and young people's mental health service was 12 weeks.

(Department for Education and Department of Health, 2017)

EDUCATIONAL PSYCHOLOGY SERVICES

Educational psychologists specifically apply their knowledge of psychology to increase the participation of children and young people in their education. In cases where mental health needs start to impact on learning, behaviour and participation in education, educational psychologists can support schools in developing specific interventions which should improve outcomes for the young person.

SCHOOL-BASED COUNSELLING SERVICES

According to the Department for Education (2016), 'counselling is an intervention that children or young people can voluntarily enter into if they want to explore, understand and overcome issues in their lives which may be causing them difficulty, distress and/or confusion' (p 6). School-based counsellors help young people to gain a better understanding of themselves and gain greater awareness of the personal resources they have at their disposal for managing specific situations. Providing access to a school-based counsellor provides more immediate support for a young person because there is no need to obtain a clinical diagnosis before a child can start to access school-based counselling. Schools may decide to refer a young person to school-based counselling for a variety of reasons, including where emotional and behavioural concerns exist or in cases of bullying. Students who experience academic pressure or other forms of stress may also benefit from counselling.

School-based counsellors tend to adopt a humanistic approach. This means that they tend to demonstrate unconditional positive regard for the young person, regardless of the situation and they help them to recognise their own strengths. Some school-based counselling services operate through a drop-in service or through an appointments-only system. There are strict professional boundaries between the counsellor and the client, and all counsellors should make these very clear to young people. School-based counsellors must make it very clear to the young person that they cannot guarantee confidentiality in cases where that person is at risk of harm. In these cases, counsellors should explain who the information will be referred to and why, and what information will be shared.

School-based counsellors can help young people to work towards goals and increase their resilience. They can support young people to work through relationship difficulties, manage their emotions, increase their motivation and self-confidence. They can reduce psychological distress in young people and they can provide support for groups of young

142

people that are at risk, including young people who identify as lesbian, gay, bisexual or transgender, young carers or those in care.

School-based counsellors can work with the young person alongside specialist support provided by CAMHS. They can also provide early intervention prior to a referral to specialist services. Some schools fund school-based counselling from Pupil Premium funding or from other funding streams in the school budget.

SCHOOL-BASED HEALTH SERVICES

School-based health services are delivered by qualified school nurses and healthcare practitioners. School-based health services can provide early intervention and can prevent problems from escalating. School-based health professionals can provide an additional layer of support in schools for young people with mental health needs. They can provide targeted interventions for a range of needs including support for managing conditions such as anxiety, depression, substance misuse or emotional health. They can teach lessons on health and wellbeing. In addition, school-based health professionals play a valuable role in enabling education colleagues to more effectively support young people with mental health needs and they can provide professional development in mental health for education staff.

SOCIAL CARE

Children's social services teams work collaboratively with schools, families and other services to ensure that children can lead safe, healthy and secure lives, so that they are able to flourish. Social care services aim to protect young people from abuse and neglect. They support vulnerable families in a variety of ways to ensure the best possible outcomes for children and young people.

Schools need to be vigilant. Young people who are being abused and neglected may demonstrate signs of poor mental health. Sudden changes to moods or behaviours should be monitored carefully. If you suspect that a mental health need has been caused by abuse or neglect, then you should discuss your concerns with the designated safeguarding lead in the school and decide whether to refer the case to the local safeguarding children's board. If the young person is in danger, then an immediate referral should be made.

Sometimes, a mental health need may not arise from abuse or neglect, but parents may require additional support in managing this need at home. In these cases, you should discuss with the parent(s) whether a referral to social care might provide an additional layer of support for the family. Some parents may become anxious of a potential referral and fear that the child will be removed from the family. You will need to reassure the parent(s) that this is extremely unlikely and will only occur if the young person is at risk of harm. Separating young people from their families is a last resort.

THE VOLUNTARY SECTOR

The voluntary sector provides vital services to support young people's mental health. Charities provide training to schools on how to support young people's mental health and some offer direct support to young people. Examples include:

Centre for Mental Health: www.centreformentalhealth.org.uk.

Young Minds: https://youngminds.org.uk.

NSPCC: www.nspcc.org.uk.

Mind: www.mind.org.uk.

Barnardo's: www.barnardos.org.uk.

Mermaids: www.mermaidsuk.org.uk.

Mental Health Foundation: www.mentalhealth.org.uk.

SIGNPOSTING FOR FURTHER SUPPORT

Parents and young people often do not know where to turn for help when they have a mental health need. Schools play a crucial role in signposting families to the services that are available in their local community and those that are available online. This can help people to get quicker support. Services are variable across the country and therefore it is not possible to provide a definitive list. Services may include those provided by the National Health Services, including:

+ general practitioners;
+ counsellors;
+ community mental health teams.

144

SUMMARY

Schools can play a significant role in developing a whole-school approach to mental health. Teachers and other education professionals can be trained in how to spot the signs of mental ill health, but they cannot diagnose a mental health disorder. This chapter has outlined the ways in which schools can work in partnership with young people and parents to give them greater participation in decision-making processes. It has outlined the roles of different professional services and provided guidance in relation to when to make a referral.

CHECKLIST

This chapter has addressed:

✓ the importance of working in partnership with young people and their parents;

✓ the different services which exist to support young people's mental health needs;

✓ the challenges associated with multi-agency collaboration.

FURTHER READING

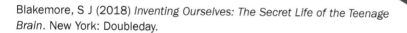

Blakemore, S J (2018) *Inventing Ourselves: The Secret Life of the Teenage Brain*. New York: Doubleday.

McDougall, T, Armstrong M and Trainor, G (2010) *Helping Children and Young People who Self-harm: An Introduction to Self-harming and Suicidal Behaviours for Health Professionals*. London: Routledge.

✚CONCLUSION

This book has emphasised the importance of reducing the stigma of mental ill health. We have stressed that schools should de-stigmatise mental health by talking about it with young people. Young people who experience mental ill health should never be made to feel guilty or ashamed because they have an illness. The role of the school is to support young people so that they can flourish.

Mental ill health that begins in childhood and adolescence can continue into adult life. Schools have a responsibility to ensure that there is parity of esteem between mental health and physical health and this attitude needs to permeate the rest of society.

Teachers have a responsibility to notice the signs of mental ill health. School leaders play a key role in ensuring that there is a positive school culture, which engenders a sense of belonging. School policies and practices should be evaluated through the lens of 'wellbeing'; where they have a detrimental impact on young people's mental health, they should be revised.

There is currently a significant emphasis by the Department for Education on character education, grit and resilience in schools. While this is not the place to define these terms, it is important to question why young people are increasingly expected to 'bounce-back' from adversity. While it cannot be denied that young people can learn a great deal from adverse experiences (such as failure), we question the role of the education system itself in contributing to mental ill health in young people. It would appear that the education system is in need of radical change. The teacher retention crisis suggests that teachers are not happy with the education system. Far too many leave the profession after three to five years. Young people are stressed, anxious and depressed. Recruitment to initial teacher training courses has been declining over several years. The emphasis on a more demanding curriculum, more challenging examinations and lack of curriculum breadth and choice results in mental ill health of young people. Some develop a poor sense of self and low confidence because the markers of educational success are too narrow. For teachers, the pressure to raise academic standards and close achievement gaps between different groups

147

of students can result in stress, anxiety, depression and burnout. The education system is toxic and has a role to play in explaining why mental ill health appears to be increasing. It is disappointing that the Green Paper (Department for Education and Department of Health, 2017) and the response to the consultation on it (Department of Health and Social Care and Department for Education, 2018) do not acknowledge the school factors that contribute to mental illness.

This book has introduced you to some common mental health needs that may be evident in young people in secondary schools. It is an introductory text and it will not have answered all your questions. It has provided you with an overview of some of the common signs of poor mental health and it has introduced you to some strategies that you can use to support young people with mental health needs.

✛REFERENCES

Anna Freud National Centre for Children and Families
www.annafreud.org

AnxietyUK
www.anxietyuk.org.uk

Association for Young People's Health (2016)
'There for You': The Role of Parents in Supporting Young People with Mental Health Problems: Results of a Survey. London: AYPH.

Banerjee, R, Weare, K and Farr, W (2014)
Working with 'Social and Emotional Aspects of Learning' (SEAL): Associations with Schools' Ethos, Pupil Social Experiences, Attendance, and Attainment. British Educational Research Journal, 40(4): 718–42.

Bond, E and Tyrrell, K (2018)
Understanding Revenge Pornography. Journal of Interpersonal Violence, 23 February: 088626051876001.

Bradlow J, Bartram, F, Guasp, A and Jadva, V (2017)
School Report: The Experiences of Lesbian, Gay, Bi and Trans Young People in Britain's Schools in 2017. London: Stonewall.

Bretherton, I (1992)
The Origins of Attachment Theory: John Bowlby and Mary Ainsworth. Developmental Psychology, 28: 759–75.

BullyingUK (nd)
What Is Bullying? [online] Available at: www.bullying.co.uk/general-advice/what-is-bullying (accessed 10 August 2018).

Child Mind Institute (2018)
Conduct Disorder Basics. [online] Available at: https://childmind.org/guide/guide-to-conduct-disorder (accessed 9 August 2018).

Children's Society (2018)
Conduct Disorder. [online] Available at: www.childrenssociety.org.uk/mental-health-advice-for-children-and-young-people/conduct-disorder (accessed 9 August 2018).

Cooper, M (2009)

Counselling in UK Secondary Schools: A Comprehensive Review of Audit and Evaluation Studies. *Counselling and Psychotherapy Research*, 9(3): 137–50.

Costa, R and Machin, S (2015)

Real Wages and Living Standards in the UK. LSE. [online] Available at: http://cep.lse.ac.uk/pubs/download/ea036.pdf (accessed 18 September 2018).

Cowie, H and Wallace, P (2000)

Peer Support in Action. London: Sage.

Department for Education (2011)

Teachers' Standards: Guidance for School Leaders, School Staff and Governing Bodies. London: DfE.

Department for Education (2016)

Keeping Children Safe in Education: Statutory Guidance for Schools and Colleges. London: DfE.

Department for Education (2017a)

Peer Support and Children and Young People's Mental Health. London: DfE.

Department for Education (2017b)

Permanent and Fixed-period Exclusions in England: 2015 to 2016. London: DfE.

Department for Education and Department of Health (2015)

Special Educational Needs and Disability Code of Practice: 0 to 25 years. Statutory Guidance for Organisations Which Work With and Support Children and Young People Who Have Special Educational Needs or Disabilities. London: DfE.

Department for Education and Department of Health (2017)

Transforming Children and Young People's Mental Health Provision: A Green Paper. London: DfE and DoH.

Department of Health and Social Care and Department for Education (2018)

Government Response to the First Joint Report of the Education and Health and Social Care Committees of Session 2017–19 on Transforming Children and Young People's Mental Health Provision: A Green Paper. Presented to Parliament

150

by the Secretary of State for Health and Social Care and Secretary of State for Education by Command of Her Majesty. Cm 9627. London: HMSO.

Education Policy Institute (2018)
Written Evidence from the Education Policy Institute, SGP0007.

Fox, C and Hawton, K (2004)
Deliberate Self-harm in Adolescence. London: Jessica Kingsley.

Gill, K, Quilter-Pinner, H and Swift, D (2017)
Making the Difference: Breaking the Link Between School Exclusion and Social Exclusion. London: Institute for Public Policy Research.

Grant, J E and Potenza, M N (2007)
Textbook of Men's Mental Health. Washington, DC: American Psychiatric Association.

Gray, S (2010)
Seen and not Heard? Living with Long-term Conditions. *British Journal of School Nursing,* 5(6): 270–1.

Healthy Young Minds
http://healthyyoungmindspennine.nhs.uk

Houlston, C and Smith, P (2009)
The Impact of a Peer Counselling Scheme in an All Girl Secondary School. *British Journal of Educational Psychology.* 79: 69–86.

House of Commons Education and Health and Social Care Committees (2018)
The Government's Green Paper on Mental Health: Failing a Generation, HC642. London: House of Commons.

House of Commons Education and Health Committees (2017)
Children and Young People's Mental Health: The Role of Education. First Joint Report of the Education and Health Committees of Session 2016-17. HC849. London: House of Commons.

House of Commons Education Committee (2018)
Forgotten Children: Alternative Provision and the Scandal of Ever Increasing Exclusions. Fifth Report of Session 2017–19, HC 342. London: House of Commons.

Lin, L Y, Sidani, J E, Shensa, A, Radovic, A, Miller, E, Colditz, J B, Hoffman, B L, Giles, L M and Primack, B A (2016)
Association Between Social Media Use and Depression Among US Young Adults. *Depression and Anxiety*, 33: 323–31.

McDaid, D, Hopkin, G, Knapp, M, Brimblecombe, N, Evans-Lacko, S and Gan, C (2017)
The Economic Case for Prevention in Young People's Mental Health: Bullying. London: London School of Economics and Political Sciences.

Morgan, C, Webb, R T, Carr, M J, Kontopantelis, E, Green, J, Chew-Graham, C A, Kapur, N and Ashcroft, D M (2017)
Incidence, Clinical Management, and Mortality Risk Following Self Harm Among Children and Adolescents: Cohort Study in Primary Care. *BMJ*, 359: j4351.

MQ: Transforming Mental Health Through Research
www.mqmentalhealth.org

National Health Service (2017)
Stepping Forward to 2020/21: The Mental Health Workforce Plan for England: A Report from Health Education England to Support the Delivery of the Five Year Forward View for Mental Health in England. London: NHS.

National Institute for Health and Care Excellence (2004)
Self-harm: The Short-Term Physical and Psychological Management and Secondary Prevention of Self-Harm in Primary and Secondary Care. Clinical Guideline CG16. London: NICE.

Okonofua, J and Eberhardt, J (2015)
Two Strikes: Race and the Disciplining of Students. *Psychological Science*, 26(5): 617–24.

Parker, C, Marlow, R, Kastner, M, May, F, Mitrofan, O, Henley, W and Ford, T (2016)
The 'Supporting Kids, Avoiding Problems' (SKIP) Study: Relationships Between School Exclusion, Psychopathology, Development and Attainment – A Case Control Study. *Journal of Young People's Services*, 11(2): 91–110.

Parsons, C, Maras, P, Knowles, C, Bradshaw, V, Hollingworth, K and Monteiro, H (2008)

Formalised Peer Mentoring Pilot Evaluation. DCSF Research Report No DCSFRR033. Paper presented at the British Educational Research Association Annual Conference, Heriot-Watt University, Edinburgh, 3–6 September 2008.

Peterson, A, Meehan, C, Ali, Z and Durrant, I (2017)

What are the Educational Needs and Experiences of Asylum-seeking and Refugee Children, Including Those who are Unaccompanied, with a Particular Focus on Inclusion? A Literature Review. Canterbury: Canterbury Christchurch University.

Public Health England (2015)

The Mental Health Needs of Gang-Affiliated Young People: A Briefing Produced as Part of the Ending Gang and Youth Violence Programme. London: PHE.

Radford, L, Corral, S, Bradley, C, Fisher, H, Bassett, C, Howat, N and Collishaw, S (2011)

Child Abuse and Neglect in the UK Today. London: NSPCC.

Refugee Council

www.refugeecouncil.org.uk

Royal Society for Public Health (2017)

#StatusOfMind: Social Media and Young People's Mental Health and Wellbeing. London: RSPH.

Royal College of Psychiatrists (2018)

Domestic Violence and Abuse. Mental Health and Growing Up Factsheet. London: RCP.

St Giles Trust (2018)

The SOS Project. [online] Available at: www.stgilestrust.org.uk/page/ sos-project (accessed 9 August 2018).

Sampasa-Kanyinga, H and Lewis, R F (2015)

Frequent Use of Social Networking Sites Is Associated with Poor Psychological Functioning Among Children and Adolescents. *Cyberpsychology, Behavior and Social Networking*, July, 18(7): 380385.

Shaw, B, Menzies, L, Bernardes, E, Baars, E, Nye, P and Allen, R (2016)

Ethnicity, Gender and Social Mobility. London: Social Mobility Commission.

Smith, N (2017)

Neglected Minds: A Report on Mental Health Support for Younger People Leaving Care. Ilford: Barnardo's.

Strand, S and Fletcher, J (2011)

A Quantitative Longitudinal Analysis of Exclusions from English Secondary Schools. University of Oxford. [online] Available at: www.education.ox.ac.uk/wordpress/wp-content/uploads/2015/02/Exclusion-from-Secondary-schools_small.pdf (accessed 18 September 2018).

World Health Organization (2018)

International Classification of Diseases. [online] Available at: www.who.int/health-topics/international-classification-of-diseases (accessed 10 August 2018).

Young Minds

https://youngminds.org.uk

✛ INDEX